A synopsis of

Occupational Medicine

F. H. Tyrer MA MRCS LRCP DIH FFOM

Consultant in Occupational Medicine
Formerly Employment Medical Adviser,
Bristol and Gloucestershire

and

K. Lee MB BS MRCS LRCP DIH FFOM

Medical Adviser, Cheshire County Council

Second edition

WRIGHT

1985 Bristol

Published by
John Wright & Sons Ltd, Techno House, Redcliffe Way, Bristol BS1 6NX, England

First edition, 1979
Reprinted, 1982
Second edition, 1985

British Library Cataloguing in Publication Data
Tyrer, F. H.
    A synopsis of occupational medicine.—2nd ed.
    1. Medicine, Industrial
    I. Title   II. Lee, Kenneth, *1926–*
    616.9′803   RC963

ISBN 0 7236 0798 2

Typeset by
Activity Ltd, Salisbury, Wiltshire

Printed in Great Britain by
John Wright & Sons (Printing) Ltd, at The Stonebridge Press, Bristol BS4 5NU

Preface to the Second Edition

In preparing this second edition we have taken heed of helpful suggestions and advice from many colleagues (including the correction of some errors in the first edition). There are three major additions to the text. The first is a chapter on Women at Work, contributed by Dr Susan Robson, which is a summary of her MFOM Dissertation. Occupational medicine in the National Health Service has been the principal growth point since the first edition was published, and we feel it merits a chapter; for contributions to this we are grateful to Dr William Benson and Dr Robin Knill-Jones. The third addition is a chapter on occupational medicine in local government services. Another major change is the omission of the whole of the text of the American Conference of Government Industrial Hygienists' publication containing their threshold limit values. Instead, we are including a note on control limits and recommended limits covered, so far, by the Health and Safety Executive Guidance Note EH40, printed herein © Crown Copyright 1984 reproduced by permission of the Controller HMSO.

We have tried to include a great deal of factual information over the wide field of occupational medicine, while at the same time preserving a discursive and readable text which conveys the concepts and philosophy of this discipline.

We acknowledge with gratitude up-to-date descriptions of occupational health services in Australia and Canada, contributed respectively by Professor David Ferguson, Director of the Commonwealth Institute of Health in the University of Sydney, and Dr Rodney May, formerly Assistant Deputy Minister in the Ontario Ministry of Labour. We also thank Dr J. A. Bonnell of the Central Electricity Generating Board for a note on ionizing radiations.

F H T   K L

Preface to the First Edition

Recent legislation, not only in the United Kingdom but in many other countries, has stimulated interest in the special health problems of work. This has meant a growing demand for specialist training. Many industrial concerns are for the first time appointing medical advisers, and these include practitioners with no previous knowledge of industrial problems. Not only these doctors, but occupational health nurses, safety officers, managements and trade unions have felt the need for information in a readily accessible form.

This book is an attempt to satisfy these requirements. Obviously, within its self-imposed limits it cannot aim to be more than a book of first reference, signposting the way to further reading and indicating the diverse fields with which occupational medicine must be concerned. The synopsis format does not encourage continuous reading, and we do not expect the book to be used in this way. However, we hope that the style and language will make it readily intelligible and useful to those without medical training who are part of the readership we aim to serve.

The toxicology section does not purport to be exhaustive, but we believe we have included most of the materials likely to be encountered in modern manufacturing industry. Naturally, there will be omissions, which will become more apparent as new technology develops; but this is inevitable in any book on the subject. We are glad to be able to include the 1977 list of threshold limit values produced by the American Conference of Governmental Industrial Hygienists.

We are particularly indebted to the Guidance Notes and other publications of the Employment Medical Advisory Service, on which we have drawn freely, and some of which we have reproduced in full, because we believe their presentation cannot be bettered. We must also acknowledge our use of the hazard data sheets in Trevethick's Environmental and Industrial Health Hazards.

Professor Alex Mair provided the initial stimulus and encouragement, and Professor C R Lowe and Dr Peter Tyrer have made valuable criticisms and suggestions on the chapters on epidemiology and psychology, respectively. To them we are especially thankful; but since the expansion of knowledge in occupational medicine depends upon the dedication and interest of relatively few doctors and experts in related disciplines, we gratefully acknowledge the help and inspiration received from all our colleagues through many years of work in this field. We must also record our appreciation of the work of our secretaries, Mrs Molly Spurrier and Mrs Sylvia Wise.

F H T   K L

Contents

Contents

Chapter 1

The Practice of Occupational Medicine

Occupational medicine in Great Britain developed from the appointment of doctors by a few companies for one of two principal reasons—to protect the company against claims at common law for industrial disease, or as part of a general paternalistic welfare policy for workers, as in William Lever's Port Sunlight and Cadbury's Bournville. Where the first aim predominated, the doctor was seen (often rightly) by workers as their antagonist—the company expert hired to deny them their rights; when the second, the emphasis tended to be on treatment, in the days before the National Health Service, and there was little or no preventive work—the doctor was rarely seen inside the factory. As in many developing countries today, what was offered was curative medicine based on the factory.

But already by 1935, when some 20 doctors met to found the Association of Industrial Medical Officers, the picture was changing. The formation of Imperial Chemical Industries, with a growing range of toxic hazards, and the increasing complexity of developing technology with its attendant new health and safety risks, led the more far-sighted employers to see that it was equally in their own interests and those of their employees to engage doctors who would study and master all serious toxicological and other health problems, know as much about the working environment as about the workers and by advice to management and regular surveillance genuinely ensure health protection for the work force.

The 1939–45 war stimulated these developments. Labour was scarce, and factories on war-work had to recruit from the less fit sections of society. A wartime Order making the appointment of doctors obligatory in factories over a certain size showed recognition of the contribution that health services could make to production. In the post-war years there was a gradual expansion of occupational health services and, along with it, acceptance of the idea that health and safety at work are in the interests of both sides of industry equally and not matters for class conflict. This implied a recognition of the doctor's impartial position and an acceptance of the ethical standards governing his work. Without any legislation to compel employers to provide a health service, by the 1960s most of the major companies in Great Britain, together with the nationalized industries, had developed services of a very high standard. Many medium-sized concerns had appointed part-time doctors, and the success of the group services initiated with Nuffield Foundation finance had proved the interest of many small companies also—although it has been the common experience of all the latter that small employers are more interested in the time-saving effect of treatment at the work place than in the preventive element.

Finally, with the inauguration of the Employment Medical Advisory Service and the passing of the Health and Safety at Work Act, the role of occupational medicine can be said to have secured universal acceptance even if its essence may still in some quarters be imperfectly understood.

Although the International Labour Office Convention of 1961 committed the signatory Governments to provision of occupational health care, each rightly interpreted the obligation in the light of its own tradition, history and special circumstances. Where general medical services are beyond the reach of large sections of the population, occupational health services will tend to be diverted to the provision of treatment, sometimes including workers' families and dependants; where there is not an effective Factory Inspectorate, occupational health doctors will often find themselves doing inspectorial work in enforcing health and safety regulations. Both are diversions; and the UK, possessing both a NHS and an experienced Factory Inspectorate, has preferred not to spell out by legislation *how* the end is to be achieved, but has made it plain what the aim is. The onus has been placed on the employer to employ the doctor and supporting staff, in preference to an attempt to provide under State control a service to industry from without; and the debate which went on for a number of years as to whether occupational medicine should form part of the NHS seems at last to have ended in the decision that it should not.

Certain basic principles can be enumerated:

1. The occupational physician is responsible for the health of the *whole enterprise*. As this depends on harmonious working between management and shop floor, he cannot be biased in favour of either side. His duty is to apply his special knowledge in this context, and when he has reached a conclusion to convey it to the proper quarter, whether it concerns management structure and practice, abuse of trade union power, or technical questions such as safe systems of working or the fitness of individuals for specific jobs.

He is in a unique position for a number of reasons—he is not competing for promotion in management, he is recognized as a repository of confidences, and even though an employee of the company, he has an independence as a member of a profession who can equally well apply his skills somewhere else.

But respect stemming from these facts is not automatic. It has to be *earned*.

2. The occupational physician is as much concerned with the working environment as with the individuals within it. Few other doctors are in a position to study aetiological factors and their effects simultaneously.

It follows that the doctor must be fully familiar with the jobs in the establishment(s) for whose health he is responsible, and must be prepared to spend time on the shop floor, observing, learning and talking to workers, managers and supervisors.

3. The doctor must be *accessible* for individual consultations. He will usually have more time for adequate listening, and counselling when required, than his colleagues in general practice or hospital practice.

As well as serving the individual, these consultations will often point to the need for investigating a work problem and be the starting point for epidemiological studies.

4. The doctor must be a *communicator* and a teacher. This implies not only health education, formal or informal, on specific occupational or more general health problems, but also making his personal contribution to management decisions, such as new production processes and their design, in which many other specialists are equally involved—the chemist, the engineer, the personnel manager, even sometimes the sales manager and the accountant. He must, however, beware the temptation to pontificate on non-medical subjects. He is

entitled to speak with authority on health; but while he is not precluded from expressing an opinion on other matters outside his field, once he steps outside it his opinion is worth no more than that of any other intelligent layman.

It is now generally accepted that the worker and his representatives must be informed of the hazards of the job and the reasons for preventive measures, as well as the results of any special tests performed. This kind of communication is an important part of the work, and should be in clear and simple language, avoiding jargon.

5. In a large occupational health team, the doctor is the coordinator, and in this sense the leader: but other kinds of specialist, in particular occupational hygienists and nurses, are masters of their own fields, and should expect full consultation about all matters affecting their specialties. From time to time they may, and should, put forward their own ideas on the general health policy. Leadership, in occupational medicine as in most other fields, does not mean autocracy. Decisions are more likely to be correct when taken after full consultation, but when there are conflicting views it is the leader who must ultimately decide how to resolve them. The occupational physician is more likely to be successful if he sees his job as leading a team than as a Napoleon with subordinates and ancillaries to do his bidding. Hence regular meetings of all medical department staff are desirable, and at them discussion should be full and frank.

In the broadest sense, the health policy of an enterprise is the responsibility of the entire management team. Here again the doctor is involved in meetings and discussions, where in addition to making his own contribution he will learn what financial, production and technical constraints have to be taken into account. An effective and realistic health policy clearly has to be framed with such consideration in mind.

RELATIONS WITH GENERAL PRACTITIONERS

There should be no rivalry or conflict between the occupational physician and the general practitioner. In the past GPs tended to look with suspicion on the doctor in industry, because they, like the workers, looked on him as the 'company doctor' who might use his position, and any information they gave him, against their patients' interests. This attitude is dying, if not dead, and has been replaced by the realization that their functions are complementary. The occupational physician has intimate knowledge of the patient's working environment and the manifestations of specific occupational illnesses; his screening procedures will from time to time reveal non-occupational conditions calling for action or investigation—chest lesions revealed by radiography, hypertension, persistent glycosuria and so on. Clearly the patient's interests require that all information of this kind should be passed to the GP. Equally the GP often knows the patient's medical history and family circumstances which may have a bearing on his fitness for his job, and if so he should inform the occupational physician—whom he knows to be bound equally with himself by the ethical code of the medical profession. (In cases of apparent ethical difficulty, when it seems desirable to acquaint management with details of matters learned from the patient or his GP, it should be remembered that this is permissible *with the patient's consent;* and most patients will give this consent if the reason it is sought, and its implications, are explained.)

Communication is always easier if the parties concerned know each other, and the occupational physician should do his utmost to meet and get to know the doctors serving the area from which employees are drawn. Visits of medical parties to the works do much to create or strengthen friendly relationships, as well as giving outside doctors valuable insight into working conditions and medical department facilities.

Laymen often ask what happens if an occupational physician and a GP disagree about, say, a patient's fitness for work. Obviously there is no rule-of-thumb answer to this, but one thing is certain: there must be *communication* in an effort to resolve it. If face-to-face discussion is not possible, the telephone is the next best medium; even the most carefully written letter can be misconstrued and arouse resentment. Moreover, many people who are prepared to be rude on paper will express their views more restrainedly in conversation, so that consensus is more easily achieved. More often than not, discussion of the case will reveal that there is in fact no conflict of view, but one side or the other has misunderstood, or been unaware of some important factor relevant to the question.

It has been well said that it is not in a patient's interest for doctors to quarrel over him.

ETHICS

The Faculty of Occupational Medicine at the Royal College of Physicians has published *Guidelines on Ethics for Occupational Physicians*. These cover the whole field of Occupational Medicine, including research. The following extracts are relevant to this chapter:

Fitness for Work

'Advice given to management about the results of a medical examination should generally be confined to advice on ability and limitations of function. Findings should only expressed in general terms, excluding clinical findings.'

Advice to Management in Respect of Individual Employees

'When there is a possibility of conflicting claims it will be found helpful to establish clearly the real needs of those who require to be serviced. Possible objections to a proposed course of action should be considered carefully and reasonable expectations should be met as far as possible. After discussion with all those concerned decisions should be made openly so that everyone knows what to expect.'

TREATMENT AT WORK

The extent to which treatment over and above emergency first aid should be given at work is a question very much bound up with these intra-professional relationships. Under the NHS, the GP is responsible for the general medical care of patients on his list, and it is he and not the works doctor who answers night calls when something goes seriously wrong. Treatment previously given to the patient at work could be significant, and if so he has a right to expect to be kept informed.

At the same time, a number of large concerns provide in their medical departments some facilities equal or superior to those in hospital—X-ray, physiotherapy and casualty facilities—and when this is so both employers and employees will fail to see why patients should undertake what may be a long and difficult journey to an overworked casualty department when in many instances they could be back on the job within half an hour after treatment at work. This consideration is particularly obvious in the case of X-rays to exclude fractures, or the insertion of sutures in minor wounds. Many minor ailments, too, can be diagnosed and treated at the outset by medical and nursing staff at work, and the judicious prescription of antibiotics for minor septic conditions may avert a spell of sickness absence. Most diseases of the skin, whether occupational or not, can be satisfactorily treated at work, and receive there more frequent supervision and change of dressings, with suitable protection, than are usually available from GP or hospital.

So the fiction that occupational health services carry out no treatment except in emergency, which was subscribed to with tongue in cheek for many years after it ceased to be true, is no longer tenable. Most GPs are now perfectly happy for works facilities to be used in this kind of treatment of their patients, provided they know the doctor in charge of them and the range of treatment available, and can have confidence that the occupational physician will use his discretion about keeping them informed.

When, however, the works doctor attends only part-time, and is a fellow GP the position is somewhat different, and the range of treatment more restricted in consequence.

PRE-EMPLOYMENT, PRE-PLACEMENT AND OTHER ROUTINE EXAMINATIONS

In the main, both management and employees now accept that the doctor has an important part to play in the place of work. But along with this acceptance, both sides of industry tend to share an unjustified belief in the preventive value of routine medical examinations of the ostensibly fit—a belief which was largely fostered by some of the arguments used in favour of a NHS before its inauguration, and to some extent strengthened by the profession itself encouraging medical mystique. The essential fallacy of this lay belief is that it over-estimates the extent and value of the information obtained by the doctor from the standard type of physical examination, and the number of disabilities detectable by it for which remedial action is possible and effective. At the same time, what is insufficiently recognized is that a factor of supreme importance in assessing an individual's fitness for a job is his psychical make-up and his motivation—something which the routine physical examination has no means of measuring, and indeed will often give no clues to, unless there is some quite extreme departure from what is generally regarded as 'normal behaviour' during the relatively short medical interview. A keen desire to do a particular job will outweigh many physical factors normally regarded as rendering a subject unfit for it, and when this exists it is a good general rule that a doctor should not stand in the way unless there are overriding reasons why he should—such as the safety of other people, or objective evidence that the patient's own estimate of his capabilities is unrealistic.

These are the considerations to be borne in mind in deciding whether pre-employment and other routine examinations should take place. In some occupations, pre-employment examinations are essential; in others they are probably desirable, but could well be simplified or modified; and in a great many others they are a sheer waste of medical man-hours which could have been better spent in more useful activities. Yet many companies beginning a health service, and many doctors entering industry for the first time, seem to decide on routine examinations as one of the first priorities—perhaps because they can produce statistical evidence of work done by the doctor. It is necessary to bear in mind the nature of the job in which the subject is, or is about to be, employed; whether the job calls for specific physical standards; the kind of relevant information which the examination could provide, and the recommendations which might be based on it. In other words, if an examination is made, its purpose is not simply to declare the subject 'fit' or 'unfit'. The words are meaningless unless qualified by an answer to the question 'Fit—for what?'

By common consent, the following kinds of occupation do call for a pre-employment examination:

1. Those which are concerned with public safety or the safety of fellow workers. Drivers of public service and heavy goods vehicles, airline pilots, navigators and food handlers, clearly come into this category, and also controllers of potentially dangerous works equipment, such as overhead crane drivers.

2. Those where the physical demands of the job call for a high standard of general fitness, for example, the police and fire services, and industrial jobs calling for physical strength and full function of limbs and special senses.

3. Those carrying a specific hazard for which a method of periodical monitoring is available. In these circumstances, the initial examination provides a base line against which subsequent developments can be checked; it then usually includes a test additional to the normal physical examination—a chest X-ray when there is a pneumoconiosis hazard; an audiogram before work in a noisy job; a blood count before exposure to radiation; a respiratory function test; and so on. In these circumstances, a full medical history is a significant part of the examination, and some applicants otherwise fit may be excluded on this alone, e.g. history of atopy before work with beryllium or isocyanates; of jaundice before work with hepatotoxic materials such as TNT, of pulmonary tuberculosis or other serious lung disease before exposure to mineral dusts. (There is no solid evidence that

such conditions render a person more susceptible to specific occupational diseases, but they may, and there is the additional consideration that if a system of the body has suffered one kind of serious insult, and recovered, it is hardly fair to subject it to the risk of a second one.)

By contrast, there is little or no point in insisting on an examination of ritual type for people entering office jobs or employment such as light assembly work which neither makes heavy physical demands nor imposes special health risks on the employee. Especially when labour turnover is high, as it tends to be in industries employing large numbers of young girls on unskilled or semi-skilled jobs, many medical man-hours can be spent in the year on largely sterile work.

Nevertheless there are many concerns where a medical examination of every new employee is a time-honoured practice, and the doctor may have to acquiesce. If this is to be done, the greater part of the examination can very well be delegated to a trained occupational health nurse who can:

Take a full medical history, using a previously prepared health questionnaire.

Measure height, weight and visual acuity, and roughly test hearing.

Take blood pressures and test urines.

Inspect skin and assess personal hygiene—condition of hair, teeth, etc.

Assess function and mobility of limbs and joints.

When this kind of screening is carried out, the nurse need refer to the doctor only those cases where the history or her findings raise doubts as to the applicant's fitness for the job envisaged. The final decision is one for the doctor, who must weigh all the known factors—which may include some which are not medical—before pronouncing on fitness for the job.

Reasons commonly advanced by employing authorities for requiring an initial medical examination are the existence of sick pay and superannuation schemes. Both rest on the fallacious belief mentioned at the beginning of this chapter—that examinations enable the doctor to make confident predictions about an employee's future work performance. This is in fact impossible, chiefly because absence attributed to sickness depends more than anything else on psychological and social factors which the doctor cannot assess. Taylor (1967, 1968) found in a continuing study of absenteeism in oil refinery workers that the pre-employment examination had no predictive value with regard to sickness absence. His study also showed that the small group of 'never sick' workers over a period of years contained no fewer than 27 per cent of registered disabled persons.

With regard to superannuation schemes, thinking tends to be muddled. The doctor is in effect being asked to predict the applicant's length of survival—which he is almost totally unable to do. But if he could, there would be no reason to exclude those likely to die or retire prematurely, since they or their dependants would receive on death or retirement benefits precisely proportionate to the amount of contributions paid. Service and benefits payable would exactly balance in the case of the employee dying on his 65th birthday, and if prediction were possible, the superannuation fund would best be protected by asking the doctor to exclude the long-livers, who would survive to draw their pensions into the 80s and 90s.

The only fair principle is to regard sick pay and pension rights as belonging to every employee found fit for engagement. Occupational physicians should attempt to educate managements out of the belief that these benefits should depend on a medical examination.

ASSESSMENT OF 'FITNESS'

The occupational physician will frequently be called upon to make decisions on an individual's fitness for the job. The question may be posed from the management side, where an employee's performance on the job has aroused doubts on his ability to continue—as for instance when someone approaching retiring age has a serious illness, or gives indications by falling standards of work that he is having difficulty in meeting the demands—or by the worker himself, who requests a change of job.

It is rare for there to be clear-cut guide lines for such cases, although for a limited range of jobs there are specific contraindications, e.g. a liability to sudden losses of consciousness will debar a man from control of potentially dangerous machinery, or from working as a scaffolder. But far more often a decision rests on a careful weighing of pros and cons, and it is in this field more than any other that the truth of the statement that medicine is an art, not a science, is illustrated. There are always lay pressures on the doctor to accept by implication the fiction that he possesses frames of reference which will enable him to give black-and-white ('either fit or unfit') answers, and that these will be based on purely medical considerations. Life is usually not like this. Medical considerations are not the only criteria governing fitness for a job, and the foreman who has watched a man at work has an opinion which may be worth as much as or more than the doctor's—his views should be sought in cases of doubt, although not necessarily always accepted. But the doctor can and should try to give an opinion on whether poor performance is likely to be caused by a health defect, and if so whether or not this is likely to be permanent. Because managers often shrink from telling an individual that he is incompetent or inadequate, a recommendation for retirement on health grounds may be seen by them as a comfortable solution; sometimes it may be the right one, but it is not one to be made simply to please management.

Decisions of this kind rest ultimately on clinical judgement, and their validity depends more on experience than on teaching. Certain principles, however, may usefully be stated:

1. No pronouncement about fitness for a job can be worth very much unless the doctor knows as much about the job as about the patient.

2. The availability of suitable alternative work and the effect on earning capacity of any change recommended are material factors. They are not necessarily decisive ones, but it is only fair to take them into account.

3. The patient's wishes must also be considered, although again they will not necessarily be decisive. Enthusiasm for a particular job can overcome physical handicap to a large extent, although overriding constraints regarding the safety of the individual and others must clearly also be taken into account. Of course there are people with no valid health reason for changing their jobs, who hope to use the doctor to secure a move. They are not difficult to identify. But in a free society, in the last analysis no one can compel a person to continue in a job he is determined to leave. Refusal to accede to such a request should be accompanied by calm and careful exposition of the reasons for the doctor's opinion. There is no reason for him to become emotionally involved, if he has given a fair and honest opinion after weighing all the relevant facts.

All organizations must have rules, but these vary in their importance and the extent to which they can safely be modified to take account of individual circumstances. Some, e.g. company rules on safety, must be regarded as absolute; but there are others, resting on tradition and precedent, of which the doctor may regard it as legitimate to recommend a 'bending' to accommodate a particular individual. The practice of medicine is based on concern for the individual human being, and in certain circumstances this may inspire a recommendation to management that an exception should be made. This is the doctor's unique contribution. And in a more general sense, since management's general health policy often has to be a compromise between what is ideally desirable and what is reasonably practicable, it is only the doctor who can advise on what kinds of compromise are permissible.

References

Health Surveillance by Routine Procedures: Health & Safety Executive, MS18.
Pre-employment Health Screening: Health and Safety Executive, MS20.
Taylor P.J. (1967) *Br. J. Ind. Med.* **24,** 93, 169.
Taylor P.J. (1968) *Br. J. Ind. Med.* **25,** 101.
Taylor P.J. (1968) *Trans. Soc. Occup. Med.* **18,** 96.

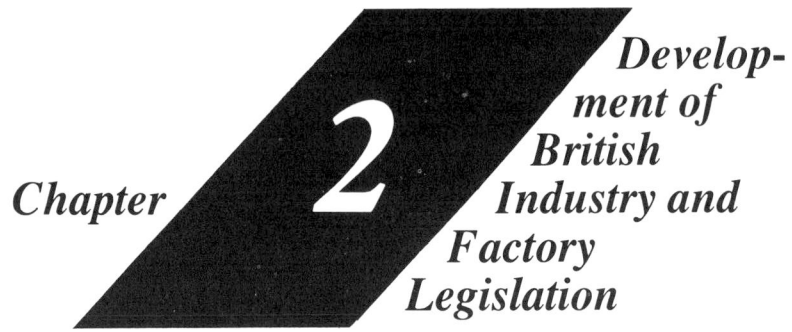

Chapter **2** Development of British Industry and Factory Legislation

The inventions of the spinning jenny (James Hargreaves, 1765), the water frame (Richard Arkwright, 1767) and the mule (Samuel Crompton, 1774–9) transformed spinning and weaving from cottage crafts to factory industries.

Mills dependent on water power (later used to raise steam) were erected along the river valleys of the Pennines and elsewhere.

Consequences

1. Workers no longer owned tools of their trade.
2. Industrial towns with housing for workers grew up around mills.
3. Traditional apprenticeship system, where each master housed, fed, clothed and trained a few apprentices applied on mass scale to children, especially from work-houses and orphanages. Personal relationship disappeared. (Poor Law authorities quick to grasp opportunity of ridding the parish of an incubus.) This often led to exploitation, overwork, malnutrition and squalor.

Legislation

Conditions at worst gradually aroused public conscience, aided by zeal of reformers.

1803 Health and Morals of Apprentices Act (Sir Robert Peel). Applied to parish apprentices in cotton mills. Hours of work limited to 12 per day; no work between 9pm and 6am. Provisions for ventilation, whitewashing of premises, clothing, religious instruction and teaching of 3Rs.

Magistrates and ministers of religion had duty to visit mills to ensure enforcement.

In fact, proved impossible to enforce.

1819 First Factories Act (Sir Robert Peel). Forbade employment of children under 9. Limited hours of work to 13½ per day for those under 16.

Again unenforceable. Enforcement left to magistrates, many of whom were themselves mill owners.

1833 Factories Act following report of Commissioners appointed at instance of Lord Ashley (later Shaftesbury).

Applied to cotton, wollen, worsted, hemp, flax, tow and silk mills.

Minimum age for starting work fixed at 9.

Limitation of hours: 48-hour week for children 9–14, 69-hour week for those 14–18.

No night work under age 18.

Two hours schooling per day for children under 11.

Four Inspectors appointed for enforcement, and doctors appointed to certify that children appeared to be not less than 9 years old. These Certifying Surgeons (later Examining Surgeons) were the forerunners of the later Appointed Factory Doctors.

1842 Mines Act. Forbade employment underground of girls, women and boys under 10—but no provision for school attendance. Mines Inspectors appointed.

1844 Factories Act. Limited hours of work of women and young persons to 12, but *reduced* minimum age for employment to 8. Limited hours to 6½ per week for children under 13. Three hours daily compulsory schooling. (Unless charity or church schools were available, employers had to provide them.)

1847 Ten-hour Act (John Fielden). Ten-hour day for women and children under 18.

1860 Mines Act. Raised age for underground employment of boys to 12—but exemption for those over 10 who produced certificates of literacy.

1864 Factories Acts Extension Act brought other industries within scope of legislation (pottery, paper staining, fustian cutting, match manufacture, cartridge manufacture).

1867 Further Extension Act to cover all industries employing over 50 people.

Workshops Regulation Act to apply to those employing less than 50—but enforcement left to local authorities.

1871 Factories Act transferred responsibility for workshops to Factory Inspectorate.

1880 Employers' Liability Act. Enabled injured workman to sue employer. Had to prove negligence.

1897 Workman's Compensation Act. Employer now liable for works accidents, regardless of negligence.

1898 Sir Thomas Legge appointed first Medical Inspector of Factories.

1906 Workman's Compensation Act extended to cover industrial diseases.

1925 Workman's Compensation Act extended list of industrial diseases.

1948 National Insurance (Industrial Injuries) Act. State took over responsibility for payment of benefit for all industrial injury and disease, regardless of consideration of negligence. Right restored to workman to sue at Common Law, in addition, recovering damages if he could prove employer's negligence. (Under Workman's Compensation Act he had to choose between receiving payments under the Act and proceeding at Common Law.)

Factories Acts were passed in 1937 (mainly a consolidating Act) and short amending Acts in 1948, 1959 and 1961.

1954 Mines and Quarries Act

1963 Offices, Shops and Railway Premises Act

1972 Employment Medical Advisory Service Act (*see* pp. 13–14)

1974 Health and Safety at Work Act (*see* pp. 14–15)

1980 Control of Lead at Work Regulations

1981 Health and Safety (First Aid) Regulations

1983 New Control Limits for Asbestos

OCCUPATIONAL HEALTH

Occupational medicine, practised through occupational health services, is concerned with:

1. The effects on work on health—occupational diseases and conditions aggravated by occupational influences.

2. The effects of health of work—matching the worker to the job, assessment of fitness for particular kinds of employment, rehabilitation and resettlement of disabled persons.

The aims of occupational health services were stated by the ILO in its OHS Recommendation 1959 (No. 112) to be:

—protection of workers against health hazards arising from the work or working conditions

—contributing to workers' physical and mental adjustment, in particular by adaptation of the work to the workers and their assignment to jobs for which they are suited

—contributing to the establishment and maintenance of the highest possible degree of physical and mental well-being

These are broad general aims, capable of interpretation in widely varying forms to meet the economic and social circumstances in each member country.

ORGANIZATION

United Kingdom

Development of occupational medicine has been chiefly through occupational health services provided *voluntarily* by larger companies and, more recently, nationalized industries. Association of Industrial Medical Officers inaugurated in 1935, with 21 founder members. 1939–45 war with emergency legislation covering factories on essential war work stimulated expansion of services, which has continued in postwar years. Provision of occupational health services paid for by employer continues to be on voluntary basis.

Group Services. Nuffield Foundation (a charitable body set up by motor magnate Lord Nuffield) has provided initial finance for setting up non-profit-making companies to provide, on a capitation fee basis, medical and nursing care at work for employees of small and medium sized firms—some on industrial estates, some in older industrial areas (Slough (1947), Harlow New Town (1955), Central Middlesex (1956), Rochdale (1962), Dundee (1962), West Midlands (1963), North of England (1960)). More recently, the West Midlands set up a satellite service at Telford, which is now self-supporting, and new services with initial finance from other sources have appeared at Milton Keynes and Newton Aycliff. Together, group services cover (1984) some 120 000 employees.

Statutory Provisions. Before 1973 statutory medical supervision was limited. Some 1300 Appointed Factory Doctors, the majority being general practitioners without occupational health training, carried out certain statutory duties including:

Examination of young people entering employment from school.

Examination of workers in processes covered by Regulations.

Investigation of gassing accidents and industrial diseases (to confirm diagnosis).

These doctors were successors of the Examining Surgeons appointed under 1833 Factories Act to certify that a child entering factory employment appeared to be over the statutory minimum age of 9.

There was also a small body of Medical Inspectors of Factories who provided specialist service for Factory Inspectorate on health matters, and collectively acquired considerable expertise in toxicology and industrial diseases. But as part of Inspectorate they tended to be associated primarily with law enforcement.

Employment Medical Advisory Service (EMAS) (Now re-named 'Medical Division of Health and Safety Executive'). Established by Employment Medical Advisory Service Act (1973), which:

Removed Medical Inspectors from Factory Inspectorate and used them as nucleus of new Advisory Service under separate administration within Department of Employment.

Abolished post of Appointed Factory Doctor (AFD) and requirement for examination of all school leavers entering industrial employment.

Recruited doctors with occupational health experience and qualifications to set up organization on regional basis, mainly full-time and covering larger areas than AFDs, up to number of 100 full-time equivalents; and subsequently a small number of Employment Nursing Advisers.

Emphasized *advisory* basis of new service, and its ready availability, without charge, with the single exception of statutory medical examinations for which the employer must pay a fee, to all interested parties. Powers and duties to investigate and advise on any health problem appearing to be related to employment, at request of:

Employer or manager;

Employee;

Trade Union;

Factory or other Inspector;

Doctor in general practice, hospital practice or public health;

Disablement Resettlement Officer;

Careers Officer;

Teacher or parent;

or on own initiative.

EMAs in the new Service took over remaining functions of AFD—statutory examinations under Regulations made under Factories Acts, investigation of gassing accidents and industrial diseases. (In recent years, much of the routine work of statutory examinations has been delegated to Appointed Doctors, with EMAs retaining a consultant rôle.)

EMAS also assumed responsibility for medical supervision of workers attending Government Employment Rehabilitation Centres and Government Training Centres (now renamed 'Skillcentres') replacing general practitioners formerly employed on sessional basis. Provided Resettlement Officers with source of medical advice in difficult cases where effect of disability on working capacity was in question; this was previously lacking when medical reports on the disabled were provided by other doctors without occupational health experience.

Statutory requirement for universal examination of school leavers entering industry replaced by selective system—somewhat complex. School Medical Officer may decide during last year at school that a child's health makes some types of employment unsuitable or undesirable, and notifies Careers Officer (on Form Y9). Careers Officer must by law be notified by employer (Form F2404) of engagement of young persons under 18 within 7 days. If Careers Officer has Y9 on same young person, both documents forwarded to EMA for investigation, at discretion, of young person and job. System has many faults, and is under review. EMA's help more likely to be valuable *before* child leaves school, and contact of all interested parties at this stage more likely to be helpful.

EMAS also responsible for initiation of and carrying out epidemiological research, either alone or in collaboration with appropriate research bodies.

It has been officially stated that EMAS is *not* a national occupational health service, and was never intended to supersede or take over the many excellent services voluntarily provided by industry and commerce. On the contrary, it works with and supplements these services and is in a position to advise on the setting up of OHS and on the quality of the existing ones. The essential difference is that EMAS is nationwide in its coverage, which extends to all industries and other fields of employment, but is essentially a consultant service, investigating specific problems; whereas the company and similar services provide *continuous* medical and nursing supervision, usually including a treatment component, for the employee groups which they cover. EMAS does not undertake any form of treatment.

Health and Safety at Work Act 1974. Set up nine-member Health and Safety Commission, Government-appointed after consultation with both sides of industry and local authorities, responsible to Secretary of State for Employment.

Commission works through three-man Health and Safety Executive which is responsible for:
Factory Inspectorate;
Mines and Quarries Inspectorate;
Alkali Inspectorate;
Nuclear Installations Inspectorate;
Explosives Inspectorate;
Employment Medical Advisory Service;
Agricultural Safety Inspectorate (from 1 Mar. 1977);
Railway Inspectorate (from 1 Apr. 1975).

Main Effects. Adds to and partially replaces exisiting legislation—Factories Act and Offices, Shops and Railway Premises Act. Most of these Acts and Regulations made thereunder remain in force, but will gradually be revised or repealed. General requirements much more detailed than any in Health and Safety at Work Act, e.g. on temperature, guarding, control of dust and fumes (Section 63).

Extends scope of health and safety legislation to *all* persons at work, including employers and self-employed—excluding only private domestic service. This added 8–9 million people to those previously covered. (In general, local authority Environmental Health Officers continue to inspect premises formerly covered by Offices, Shops and Railway Premises Act. They have liaison with the Factory Inspectorate.)

Aims not only to safeguard people at work, but also others affected by work processes, e.g. by emission of noxious or offensive substances, or mishaps with explosive or inflammable material.

Duties of Employers. General duty to safeguard health, safety and welfare of employees. Provision of safe systems of working—including use, handling, storage and transport of articles and substances.

Provision of a written statement on health and safety policy and publicizing this to employees.*

Arrange for election by employees of safety representatives, and for setting up of safety committees.

Conduct the undertaking with due regard for the health and safety of persons *not* employed, and in prescribed circumstances give them information about such aspects of the work as may affect their health and safety.

(Many of these clauses are qualified by the words 'so far as reasonably practicable').

Duties of Manufacturers. Manufacturers includes those who design, manufacture, supply, erect or install any article, plant, machinery, equipment or appliances for use at work, or manufacture, import or supply any substance for use at work.

They are required to:

Ensure that design and construction is safe and without health risk when properly used.

Carry out testing and examination to this end.

Give adequate information about testing, proper use and any necessary conditions for safe use.

Conduct or arrange research directed at eliminating or minimizing health and safety risks of the equipment or material.

Ensure safe erection or installation.

Duties of Employees. An employee must:

Take reasonable care for the health and safety of himself and others who may be affected by his acts or omissions at work.

Cooperate with the employer in the carrying out of any duty or requirement designed for health and safety.

Powers of Inspectors

To enter premises at any reasonable time.

To take along 'any unduly authorized person' and take measurements, photographs and recordings.

*Enterprises with less than 5 employees may be exempted from this requirement.

To take samples and require information relevant to the investigation.

To issue prohibition orders, or improvement orders calling for rectification within a specified time of faults, on employers operating a process with a risk to health or safety.

To prosecute for breaches of statutory regulations.

There is also a duty to disclose relevant information about their health and safety to employees, and to assist in keeping them adequately informed on these matters.

Occupational Health Services in UK. Most of the largest companies in manufacturing industry, and an increasing number of those in retail trade, now provide occupational health services. So do the nationalized industries—coal, railways, electricity, gas, steel and docks.

Many other companies employ part-time doctors, but these are usually general practitioners without occupational health qualifications, and by no means all are in fact practising occupational medicine—a number are concerned only with treatment of work injuries and illness and minor ailments occurring at work. But it is estimated that about 85% of companies employing 34% of the working population provide no service other than statutory first aid cover.

Specialised services to handle the problems of divers and others working on North Sea oil installations are a recent development, and there is a small but growing number of private consultants. Most universities and polytechnics provide student health services, and in some instances, but probably not the majority, these also provide an occupational health service for university staff.

There are about 1000 doctors practising occupational medicine full-time and 2000 part-time, and about 9000 nurses. (Report of House of Lords Select Committee on Science and Technology. Session 1983–84: Occupational Health & Hygiene Services. 99-I.)

Occupational health services for hospital and local authority employees are a comparatively recent development following the Tunbridge Report (1968. The Care of the Health of Hospital Staff). There are between 200 and 300 such services at the time of writing (1984). A number of English regions have appointed full-time consultants, as have all but one of the Scottish regional health authorities.

DHSS Health Notice (HN(82) 33) contains guide-lines on the functions of these services—selective pre-employment screening, maintenance of records, advice on immunizations and environmental conditions, guidance and health assessments. (*See also* Chapter 11 on hazards of hospital employment).

Relationship between Occupational Health Services and the National Health Service. The National Health Service was set up in 1948 to care for the nation's health, both in the field of prevention and therapeutics. Fairly early in its life the treatment services demanded such a high priority that preventive services were omitted or at least dealt with in a very summary way. It was not until the reorganization of 1974 that the public health services were absorbed into the National Health Service.

In 1951 the Dale Committee enquired into industrial health services and came to the view that voluntary services, with the existing statutory services, could not by themselves be expected to be adequate for the whole of industry, especially in regard of the smaller firms. The Committee thought that some kind of comprehensive provision should eventually be made for both industrial and non-industrial occupations. This recommendation was never taken up by the Government.

The BMA set up a working party (Alexander Report) in 1961 and this, together with the Porritt Committee which reported in 1962, urged the Government to set up a comprehensive occupational health service under the NHS Area Health Boards. The Report stated 'the National Health Service should be responsible through Area Health Boards for running all medical services including preventive and social health services and occupational health services covering industry and commerce.' The Porritt Committee suggested that the NHS should be required to provide services for those firms without a service and which were unlikely ever to establish one for themselves; again there was no response from the Government.

In 1968 the Tunbridge Committee reported on the care of hospital staff. The last sixteen years has been a very fragmented and, on the whole, a very indifferent development.

In May, 1970 the Secretary of State for Employment and Productivity set up a Committee to enquire into the provisions made for the safety and health of persons in employment (excepting transport workers who were covered by other provisions) and to consider whether any changes were needed. Lord Robens was the chairman of this committee which reported in 1972. This report led to the Health and Safety at Work Act 1974. The Robens Committee was critical of some of the existing industrial medical services, where it was thought that many doctors were spending too much time on the treatment of patients, thus duplicating the facilities which should be provided by the NHS. The Report estimated that about one-third of the time of the Group Services was taken up by casualty work and treatment. The Report also pointed out that occupational health was a combination of various disciplines requiring the skills of the chemist and engineer, as well as a knowledge of the medical specialist. An occupational health service was not synonymous with general medical care provided at the point of occupation. It does not imply the need to have a doctor at every sizeable factory. It was clear that the Robens Committee regarded the development of the Employment Medical Advisory Service as a foundation of occupational medicine for the country and it did not recommend that the Government should involve itself further in the provision of an occupational health service.

By 1983 occupational health services were still fragmented and unequal.

The House of Lords Select Committee on Science and Technology conducted an enquiry under the chairmanship of Lord Gregson into the future provision of occupational health and hygiene services. This report (Gregson Report) was published in December 1983.

The Committee addressed itself to the following questions:

1. Is supervision of occupational health and hygiene services in industry adequate?

2. What kinds of service should be offered; how best might they be developed?

3. Should the State assume responsibility for comprehensive industrial health services and, if not, which body should be expected to undertake initiatives in this field?

The Committee also considered the adequacy of funds for research and the effects of cuts in university spending and a growing reluctance on the part of employers to sponsor candidates for education and training.

The Committee reviewed the existing services. A high proportion of British workers work in small firms and so the absence of occupational health services is all the more serious. 67% of the 12½ million employed in services industries, 43% of 9 million employed in production industries and 57% of 21½ million employed in all industries and services work in units employing fewer than 200 people; that is firms which usually have no medical or nursing service except, in a few instances, a doctor being on call.

Table 3.1. Distribution of full and part-time Membership of the Faculty of Occupational Medicine—by industry

Industry	Full time	Part time	Employees/doctor
Construction	2	2	327 000
Insurance and banking	3	3	290 000
Distributive trades	10	2	240 000
Agriculture, forestry and fishing	4	—	86 000
Shipbuilding	2	1	54 000
Mechanical engineering	8	10	53 000
Professional and scientific	78	48	35 000
Food, drink, tobacco	26	21	16 000
Transport	96	13	13 000
Gas, electricity, water	25	8	11 000
Public administration and defence	125	37	10 000
Chemical industry	61	2	5 000
Mining and quarrying	83	13	4 000
HM Forces	147	—	2 200
All	856	275	21 000

The ratio of doctors to workers varies considerably from one industry group to another, for example coal and petroleum products, mining and quarrying, chemical manufacturing and metal manufacture are far better provided for than ship building, engineering or construction industries. Clearly there are factors other than need which determine the provision of occupational health services.

In the National Health Service a survey in 1981 showed that there were 370 doctors employed in occupational medicine, only 12 of whom were full time. Only 13% of these doctors had a specialist qualification in occupational health. There were 592 nurses employed full time, of whom 37·6% held the occupational health nurses certificate.

The Committee's conclusion from all this evidence was that large scale manufacturing undertakings, on the whole, make adequate provision although there is a very wide variation. Small firms make very little or no provision. Government employees, whether civil or military, are well provided for. The employees in the NHS have an extensive but rather rudimentary service.

The Committee consider that extension of the occupational health services was necessary, especially in the medium and smaller sized firms which had a much less satisfactory provision than the larger undertakings. The Committee attached considerable importance to preventive medicine and pointed out that early detection of hazards at work and the timely adoption of preventive measures would not only alleviate the individual's suffering; they would lighten financial burden which sickness imposes upon the State.

The Committee took the view that occupational health should be regarded as an integral part of the primary care of patients. An individual spends so much of his life at work that occupational medicine should play a more prominent part in the primary service which is available to him. Both general practice and occupational medicine are concerned, after all, with the same patients. As much of occupational health work is now done by general practitioners and nurses, the Committee proposes that these practitioners should have the appropriate qualifications.

The Committee concluded that occupational health services should continue to be provided on a private basis founded largely by employers in reflection of their general duty under Section II of the Health and Safety at Work Act. However, some increase in Government support will be necessary. The Committee were reluctant to recommend a statutory requirement as it would create a demand for trained personnel greater than the supply available, it would impose unwelcome and sudden additional costs to industry, it might provoke hostility and resentment where co-operation and sympathy are crucial, it would lead to bureaucracy, and the Committee doubted whether statutory arrangements would be sufficiently flexible for the widely varying needs. The Committee favoured the voluntary approach by suggesting a code which would lay down in general terms the qualifications of personnel, the provision of appropriate facilities, the working relationships between personnel, management and unions, and the control of the services. Some incentives could be offered to employers by allowing tax relief on capital expenditure and a reduction of insurance premiums. Failure to observe the code may well be invoked in the Courts as evidence in actions for negligence.

It was evident from the survey that to spread occupational health services to the medium and smaller firms there should be an increase in the number of general practitioners doing part-time occupational health work. These doctors should have appropriate training (*see* pp. 20–21). The many nurses employed in occupational health should also receive adequate training (*see* p. 21).

The Committee recommended that EMAs should do far more advisory and research work and not be involved in so many statutory examinations. There should be a return to the appointed factory doctor system for these routine tasks.

Functions of the Occupational Physician
Advisory. Advice to management on all conditions affecting employees' health, including:
  Prevention of occupational disease;
  Study of sickness absence;
  Working conditions affecting employees' physical and mental health and morale;
  Medical aspects of legislation about employment;
  Medical aspects of welfare services.
Clinical. Carrying out suitable pre-employment or pre-placement examinations when appropriate.
  Surveillance by appropriate means of employees exposed to specific hazards.
  Assessment of fitness for particular jobs after illness or injury with view to rehabilitation and resettlement.
  Supervision of nursing and first aid services.
  First aid treatment of injuries and illness at work and (usually by agreement with local GPs and hospital services) continued treatment of some conditions.

(The extent of follow-up treatment will depend to a great extent on the facilities available. It is often expedient and in everyone's interest to avoid loss of working time by treatment of these conditions which can readily be treated at work; but clearly professional courtesy and the patient's interest require that his regular medical attendant should be informed of anything done which is significant from the point of view of his subsequent health.) (*See* p. 5.)

Health Education. Opportunities frequently arise for individual health education arising from consultations. Talks to working groups about particular occupational hazards may from time to time be undertaken. These are preferably short and informal.

Familiarity with the working environment is essential for the effective practice of occupational medicine. Opportunities for *voluntary consultation* are also important—often provide first indication of health hazard.

Training. The Faculty of Occupational Medicine at the Royal College of Physicians, London, prescribes training and qualifications in this specialty. After three years of general professional training, following registration, the trainee will undertake a four-year programme of specialist training. In the early part of the programme the trainee can sit the examination for associateship of the Faculty (AFOM). On completion of four years' training in an approved post, and after the acceptance of a dissertation which can be submitted during the training period, the trainee is awarded membership of the Faculty (MFOM).

To obtain specialist registration the trainee has to have held a post, or a number of posts, which have been approved as training posts by the Joint Committee on Higher Medical Training (JCHMT).

Although attendance at a formal course of training is not mandatory, it is strongly advised. The London School of Hygiene and Tropical Medicine, Keppel St., London WC1E 7HT organizes courses for the MSc in Occupational Health (9 months full-time or 2 years part-time) and for the Diploma in Industrial Health (3 months full-time); particulars from Registrar. Other full-time courses may be held at The Wolfson Institute of Occupational Health, University of Dundee and The Institute of Occupational Medicine, Edinburgh.

Part-time training by a day-release scheme lasting two years is given by the Department of Occupational Health, University of Manchester, Stopford Building, Oxford Road, Manchester.

The British Life Assurance Trust (BLAT) has sponsored a distance learning project for occupational medicine. The course, consisting of booklets and tapes, is supplemented by seminars which may be attended either in person or by arranging telephonic links. These courses are particularly suitable for trainees who are at some distance from a University Department. Details can be obtained from Mr Ted Stephenson, Department of Occupational Health, Manchester University.

The AFOM examination is designed both as a step towards specialist accreditation and as a demonstration of knowledge and competence in its own right. It would be useful to medical practitioners who have only a part-time interest in occupational medicine and do not wish to proceed to full specialist status. The Gregson Report (*see* p. 17) considered that the AFOM was too high a standard for many of the general practitioners who held only part-time appointments in occupational medicine. It was proposed that there should be a shorter course, arranged at provincial centres, which would suit their particular needs. It is intended that the course syllabus of thirty hours tuition should have the approval of the Faculty and be recognized by the Medical Division of the Health and Safety Executive.

Joint Committee on Higher Medical Training. This committee contains representatives of the Royal Colleges of Physicians and Surgeons, Royal College of Pathologists, Faculty of Community Medicine, Association of Clinical Professors of Medicine, Conference of Postgraduate Deans and specialist associations, plus observers from Government Departments.

Nurses. The Royal College of Nursing awards on Occupational Health Nursing Certificate after approved training and examination. Evidence of an approved standard of general education, a personal interview, an entrance test paper and professional references are required before admission to the examination.

Courses may be either full-time, or part-time day release for those already employed in occupational health nursing. Both comprise not less than 320 hours' tuition by approved lecturers, spread over two academic terms if full-time, or 65 days in 5 academic terms of day release.

The examination consists of three parts:

1. Periodic assessment throughout the course, entailing the submission of 5 pieces of work, 30% of marks.

2. A final written examination (3 hours), 40% of marks.

3. Special study on a topic of the student's own choice, demonstrating an understanding of occupational health nursing (6000–8000 words), 30% of marks.

The College has also recently started a course for an occupational health nurse practice award, which is intended to increase the nurse's competence in her day-to-day work. Training is of a practical nature, lasting 120–140 hours, and Enrolled Nurses are eligible. There is also an Occupational Health Nursing Appreciation Course, which is *not* intended to prepare nurses to work in industry but as part of general nurse training, or for health visitors and district nurses.

Copies of the syllabus for all these courses and a list of approved centres offering training for the Occupational Health Nursing Certificate may be obtained from the Director of Education, Institute of Advanced Nursing Education, Royal College of Nursing, Henrietta Place, London, W1M 0AB.

Employers' Liability (Compulsory Insurance) Act 1969. Responsibility for administration transferred to Health and Safety Executive 1 April, 1975.

Requires employers, other than public bodies, to take out and maintain approved insurance policies with authorized insurers against bodily injury or diseases sustained by employees in course of employment.

Since extended to cover employment on offshore installations.

W. Europe

European Economic Community (EEC) countries all subject to ILO Recommendation (No. 112, 1959) on occupational health services but have not all thought it necessary to introduce legislation. Belgium and the Netherlands both require employers in enterprises of defined size to provide health services. France has had since 1946 legislation embracing most fields of employment, but the emphasis is mainly on pre-employment and routine examinations, and treatment is specifically excluded; on the other hand, much emphasis is placed on rehabilitation and resettlement.

The German Federal Republic passed a Safety at Work Act in 1973. This contains detailed provisions requiring all employers to appoint medical advisers and safety engineers. The numbers of hours per year to be devoted by each to the work is calculated on a formula taking into account the numbers employed and the nature of the employment. Works safety committees and workers' safety representatives must be appointed. Doctors undertaking the work must produce evidence of attendance at a course in occupational medicine. It is estimated that 9000 doctors with this training will be needed. There are Academies of Occupational Medicine in Berlin and Munich.

Most, but not all, member countries now provide similar training courses in occupational medicine. Representative committees within the EEC are working towards a 'harmonization' of occupational medical practice and standards in member countries: but progress will necessarily be slow.

In other European countries—Austria, Norway, Spain, Sweden, Switzerland and Portugal—occupational health services are provided by major companies, and in both Norway and Sweden both Government and trade unions take an active interest.

Japan

Japanese legislation on health and safety at work is broadly on the same lines as that of Western Europe. The Ministry of Labour, which is responsible for this and all other aspects of regulation of employment, was established in 1947 as an offshoot of the former Welfare Ministry. New legislation on factory inspection and security of employment was introduced about the same time, as were laws on Workmen's Compensation and Unemployment Insurance. Trade unions were legalized, and rules for labour relations were formalized. The unions are company-based rather than industry-based. They have statutory representation on a number of national bodies concerned with labour relations, and also on works safety committees.

An Industrial Health and Safety Law, passed in 1972 and amended in 1975, 1977, 1980 and 1983, covers current employment conditions. It defines the responsibilities of the employer for health and safety at work, and empowers the Minister to make regulations for particular industries on matters such as accident prevention, the appointment of safety and health supervisors, and of industrial physicians, and the setting up of safety committees. There is a system of certification of machinery before use, and of periodic inspection and maintenance. The manufacture of some chemicals is forbidden and of others permitted only under controlled conditions. In certain industries and on specified processes, medical examinations are compulsory—but workers have the right to opt for examination by a physician other than the company physician. The duties of the 'industrial health consultant' are defined as to 'make diagnosis of health in the work-place and give guidance based on such diagnosis for the improvement of the level of health of workers' and a statutory examination must be taken by doctors wishing to undertake this work. Only doctors so qualified are entitled to work in industry. Medical advisers are attached to local Labour Standards Offices; they are part-time, and visit work-places to investigate specific problems on request. The law provides for research and epidemiological surveys.

Communist Countries

In general, the Communist countries of E. Europe tend to base general medical services, covering employees and their families and dependants, on the factory or place of employment. It is hence difficult to judge what percentage of the medical staff described as employed by a particular enterprise is in fact practising occupational medicine as opposed to general therapeutic services.

Enquirers seeking specific information about a particular country should apply to that country's Embassy.

'Third World'

Many recently independent and developing former colonial countries have established university departments or institutes of occupational health, and some large companies provide health services for employees and their dependants. Most of these countries are poor, and in many of them both general medical services and public health services are at a rudimentary level; hence factory health services, when they exist, provide all three. Occupational health services depend to a large extent on an infra-structure of basic health care, and in countries which lack such provisions as a safe drinking water supply and sewage disposal systems, protection against specific occupational risks cannot be a very high priority.

United States of America

Occupational Safety and Health Act 1970 established National Institute for Occupational Safety and Health within Department of Health, Education and Welfare. This is a Federal agency responsibility for: occupational safety and health standards; research, education and training.

The Act requires employers to provide a work-place free from recognized hazards likely to cause death or serious harm to employees: covers industrial, agricultural and construction workers. Previously only State-enforced 'consensus standards' and federal regulations applied only to Federal employer.

Recommendations made to appropriate Government Department which is responsible for legislation and enforcement. Three research centres (principal laboratories in Cincinnati, Ohio) and 10 Regional Offices which conduct special surveys and provide consultative services.

Secretary of Labor responsible for promulgating consensus and established Federal safety standards.

NIOSH produces 'criteria documents' giving recommended standards of exposure to occupational hazards and lists of Threshold Limit Values, with methods of control. Produced in 1971 list of 8000 substances known to be toxic, with TLVs—available from US Government Printing Office, Washington, DC.

National Advisory Committee contains employers, unions and occupational health and safety practitioners.

Federal Inspectors have right to inspect, investigate and enforce standards, and employees may request an inspection. There are 1200 of them.

Individual States have their own legislation, but many have drawn up plans similar to the Federal Act. Federally-approved schemes qualify for up to 50% Federal grant, and States receive up to 90% of the cost of surveys to discover needs and develop plans. In December 1975 23 States were operating federally approved plans.

The American Board of Preventive Medicine has recognized occupational medicine as a specialty since 1955. Postgraduate training includes 1 year's approved residency followed by 2 years of graduate study in preventive and occupational medicine.

The Industrial Medical Association is the national professional organization for physicians engaged in occupational medicine. It has 30 component societies in USA, publishes Journal of Occupational Medicine monthly, and provides a number of services to members as well as organizing annual conferences.

Canada

Canada is a country in which industrial development stems directly from the exploitation of its vast natural resources—timber, coal, land crops, stock raising—and later nickel, asbestos, ferrous ores, fishing, hydroelectric power, potash, uranium, oil and natural gas. Prior to Confederation there was the traditional pattern of excessively long working hours, unsafe factories and workshops, crowded working conditions, child labour and low wages. Development of such a vast country—most of which is near arctic for much of the time—resulted in the establishment of separately governed 'provinces' loosely held together by a 'federal' body. While Confederation greatly improved the picture, the individual establishments continued and many remain to this day. Each province maintains its own medical and nursing 'regulatory' and disciplinary bodies. Reciprocity of licences to practice is still not universal.

Canada now has an extensive programme covering occupational health, medicine, nursing, occupational hygiene, etc. Diploma, Certificate and Masters' programmes are offered at many universities and through Community Colleges. There is Board Certification, comparable to that in the USA, through a national board (for physicians) and in 1984 after some five years of negotiation and deliberation, The Royal College of Physicians and Surgeons of Canada now recognizes occupational medicine as a specialty in its own right. There is now certification on a national basis for occupational health nurses (an extension of the OHNC programme for nurses first developed for nurses in 1974 through Grant Macewen College in Alberta).

Each province now has its own occupational health programme, and Occupational Health Services are also available through National Health and Welfare and Labour Canada to serve the federal employees scattered throughout the provinces. Services are also provided to employees of agencies coming under federal control—certain mining operations, docks, transport etc. Radiation health is also generally under federal control with provinces acting as agents in implementing the legislation.

The federal government has also established a national council (Canadian Council for Occupational Health and Safety) to co-ordinate Occupational Health and Safety activities across the country. Each province has representation from management, government and labour and assists in identifying needs, developing policy guides, etc.

There is also an Associated Canadian Centre for Occupational Health and Safety which provides for practical needs—technical services, information systems, international liaison, has established a data base and promotes (with federal financial assistance) research into occupational health and safety.

While generally it may be considered that Canada was for many years (other than in Ontario and Quebec) somewhat tardy in recognizing needs and supplying services and education, it has caught up fast in the last decade and has a highly credible programme in all areas.

Legislation is somewhat in advance of many English-speaking countries and is aimed more at prevention and problem solving than at rigid regulatory systems. It is generally based on the principles of the Right to Know, the Right to Participate in Remedial Programmes and the Right to Refuse Unsafe Work. Most provinces have an independent Government Advisory Committee with membership drawn from management, labour and the public at large and charged with the duty of advising Government on all aspects of occupational health and safety.

For those who wish to make contacts or have more detailed information, a useful resource document is the CORPUS Occupational Health & Safety Management Handbook 1985 obtainable from Corpus Information Services, 1450 Don Mills Road, Ontario M3B 2X7.

Australia

In Australia's federal system, laws and regulations on occupational health and safety are devised and administered separately by each of the six states and two territories. Law and practice on health and safety in the workplace have in the past been firmly separated at federal and state level and in industry—occupational health in Ministries of Health, and safety in Ministries of Labour. Within this dichotomy, some uniformity in practice has been achieved by means of state and territory membership of national committees; and by the generation, under their aegis, of model legislation, standards, codes of practice and guides which tend to be adopted into regulations or otherwise achieve the force of law.

Most states and territories have, in the past ten years, created new occupational health and safety legislation usually based on, if not going as far as, the United Kingdom's Health and Safety at Work etc. Act of 1974. In the same period, there has been a progressive move for government divisions of occupational health in each state and territory to be taken over by Ministries of Labour. Major changes at the national level were initiated in 1983 after the election of a Federal Labour Government. Changes currently being developed (in 1984) include a National Occupational Health and Safety Commission, answerable to the Minister of Employment and Industrial Relations; a National Occupational Health and Safety Office in that ministry; an Environment Contaminants Authority in the Department of Home Affairs and the Environment; and a National Institute of Environmental and Occupational Health and Safety in the Department of Health.

Over half (56%) of workers in manufacturing in Australia are in factories employing less than two hundred people. Only the large corporations employ in-plant health professionals. However, manufacturing establishments represent less than a third of all sources of employment, and many occupational health professionals work in service and government industry. The numbers of such professionals employed full-time (in 1984) have been increasing rapidly. As some indication, the Australian and New Zealand Society of Occupational Medicine in that year had a membership of about 470 (including New Zealand); the new Australian College of Occupational Medicine had about 230 members; about 2000 nurses, the great majority untrained in occupational health, work in industry, private and public; the Australian Institute of Occupational Hygienists had 60 members; and the Ergonomics Society of Australia and New Zealand had 350 members in Australia. There has been a rapid growth also in the numbers of private consultants in occupational medicine; and in private industrial clinics, which started as clinical (work injury) services and progressively are becoming more preventively oriented.

A further recent trend has been towards corporate occupational health and safety groups in large government and private establishments, which often include physicians, hygienists, nurses, ergonomists, physiotherapists, and safety engineers in a team. Several multidisciplinary private consulting groups have sprung up. Industries are also employing health and safety managers in place of, or in addition to, traditional safety officers. Among their functions is to administer the workplace health and safety committees now being appointed increasingly, particularly in New South Wales where such committees are required under its Occupational Health and Safety Act of 1983. However, most workers get no health cover at the workplace; what cover exists is still mainly provided by general practitioners.

Except in Queensland where nurses are required for workplaces of over 300 people, there are no statutory obligations to provide occupational health services, but legislation calls for periodic examination of workers exposed to certain hazards such as lead, asbestos and some solvents. State divisions of occupational health undertake biological monitoring and visit workplaces on request.

The range of activities of in-plant services depends partly on hazard and distance from city services. In addition to accepted screening and preventive activities, most services now take on rehabilitation and health promotion, including alcohol programs. Minor treatment including first aid is usually undertaken to the extent that referral to other community services is unnecessary, or that it enables a worker to complete a shift.

Israel

A Safety at Work Act and regulations made thereunder provide the basic legislation on occupational health. This covers general welfare provisions as well as specific hazards.

A national insurance scheme ensures benefits for all occupational diseases and injuries (50 diseases are scheduled). Sickness insurance is voluntary on the worker's part, but employers pay compulsory contributions. Occupational health services are financed by insurance funds.

The Kupat-Holim (Worker's Sick Fund Medical Insurance) is a nationwide autonomous medical insurance sponsored by the General Federation of Labour which provides comprehensive medical services in its own clinics (rural and urban) health centres, institutions and hospitals to roughly 72% of the total population of Israel. The remaining 28% are covered by several smaller insurance schemes which usually make use of the K. Holim when occupational health is concerned.

Organization. The Ministry of Labour and Welfare is responsible for enforcement of legislation. The Inspectorate includes two Medical Inspectors and an Environmental Health Laboratory.

There is an Occupational Safety and Hygiene Institute attached to the Ministry, with a Board of Management representing employers, employees and Government. Its activities are mainly educational.

Occupational health services run by the Workers' Sickness Insurance cover the whole working population. Sixty doctors and 60 nurses operate in 15 regional departments. In addition, a few plants have their own staff. The Society of Occupational Physicians has 80 members, and there are 100 occupational health nurses.

Workplaces are visited for the investigation of problems, and on a routine basis. There are Regional Dispensaries with full diagnostic facilities to which workers are referred for a consultant opinion. Laboratory facilities for environmental and biological tests exist at the Institute of Occupational Health at Tel-Aviv.

Training. Undergraduate teaching and occupational health research are undertaken at all four of the country's medical schools—the Hebrew University of Jerusalem, Tel-Aviv, Beer-Sheva and Haifa. Postgraduate training is done at the first two of these.

International Commission on Occupational Health

(Formerly Permanent Commission and International Association on Occupational Health.)

Founded in 1906 in Milan as international scientific society. Organizes triennial international congress on occupational health and has a number of committees on specialized topics.

Occupational physicians, hygienists and nurses eligible for membership.

Sources of General Information

TUC Centenary Insitute of Occupational Health, London School of Hygiene and Tropical Medicine, Keppel Street, London WC1E 7HT, Tel. 01-636-8636. Provides an information service on all aspects of occupational health.

Medical Adviser to the TUC (Dr R. Owen), Congress House, Great Russell Street, London WC1B 3LS, Tel. 01-636-4030. Advice to unions on occupational health problems.

International Labour Office, 87–91 New Bond Street, London W1Y 9LA, Tel. 01-499-2084. London office of Geneva-based ILO which offers advice on occupational health.

Health and Safety Executive, Information point, St. Hugh's House, Stanley Precinct, Bootle, Merseyside L20 3QY. Information about safety and health legislation.

National Occupational Hygiene Service, 12 Brook Road, Fallowfield, Manchester M14 6UH, Tel. 061-224-9191. Independent assessment of environmental problems, including biological monitoring.

Institute of Occupational Medicine, Roxburgh Place, Edinburgh EH8 9SU, Tel. 031-667-5131.

Bibliography

Occupational Health: *A Guide to Sources of Information.* (Ed. Gauvain) 1974, London, William Heinemann Medical Books.

Health and Safety Commission. Report 1976–7. London, HMSO.

Occupational Health Nursing Practice (Ed. Cynthia Harris) 1984. Bristol, Wright.

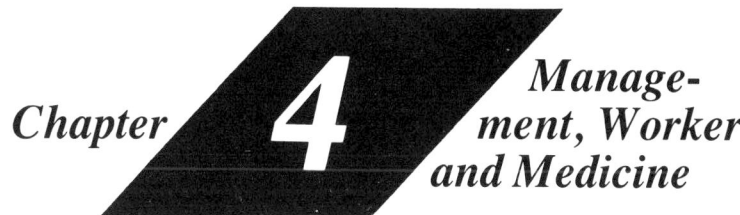

Chapter 4 — Management, Worker and Medicine

MANAGEMENT

Before the Industrial Revolution family businesses were set up with small initial capital, the owner had intimate control, he lived near the factory and he often developed a benevolence to local society. There were close personal contacts, a single line of authority, quick decisions and in these small concerns everyone saw the end result of their labours. With prevailing high unemployment and poverty, the threat of dismissal was a very powerful disciplinary factor.

With the development of costly machinery and mechanical power in the 19th century, joint stock companies were formed and few family businesses survived. Owners became remote from the work and there has been the evolution of the career manager. Growth of business has led to the functionalization of management and the use of techniques of management measurement and control.

Possible Inefficiencies

Unless active measures are taken to ensure coordination, the organization becomes inefficient through:

Increasingly remote control from the top;
Loss of personal contact;
Loss of sense of belonging;
Difficult communications;
Administration confusion and overlap;
Proliferation of paper work;
Uncoordinated specialization;
Inter-departmental rivalries;
Status-seeking;
Loss of the competitive edge of cost-consciousness;
External intervention by government control, which can impair dynamism in management.

Positive Management

There should be a clear definition of the purpose of the business, and of each section.

The management philosophy must recognize human values and social conditions.

The work people must feel that they belong to the business, and have a definite contribution to make.

There must be a sound system of communication both ways.

Top management should be confined to policy decisions, and not become involved in day-to-day routine.

As the social environment and the needs of industry change, so management should anticipate change, define alterations to the organization, and channel energy into useful work, not into frustration. It is important to select and train managers.

These points are fundamental to good management, and are stated baldly and concisely; but a little amplification may help to bring them to life. The *purpose* of the undertaking is essentially the provision of goods and services, which are the material wealth financing every national activity. This truth is often not appreciated by the shop-floor worker, who all too often has been led to believe that the only purpose is to make profits for shareholders (even when in fact no profits are made, or when the industry is nationalized and running at a loss). 'The Government' which in fact has no funds except what is derived by taxation from industry and its employees, is seen as the provider of welfare and other benefits. He tends therefore to adopt an attitude of caring only about his own pay packet and to be indifferent to the performance of the enterprise. The conveyance of this information to him regularly, down the management line through supervisors, is the best way of ensuring that he feels personal involvement in a worthwhile enterprise. This is what leadership means. Progressive managements ensure that all levels of management and supervision are kept fully briefed on company policy and performance, and recognize that it is their job to pass it on.

Britain has a number of highly successful enterprises applying this policy in practice. The poor performance of others, and their poor record in labour relations, reflects a failure of management to do this, with consequent alienation of the rank-and-file worker.

Top management must itself be convinced that the points listed mean precisely what they say, and that their implementation is not something to be remembered occasionally, but a continuous process which is an integral part of the day-to-day business of running the organization.

In recent years it has become the practice in some companies for communication to pass down the line from higher management to shop stewards, bypassing the supervisor. This is a recipe for chaos; the shop steward's function is to represent the work force, but the supervisor's is to represent the management in the process of two-way communication.

Not everyone is born with the qualities of leadership; but they can be inculcated by training, and successful management depends on training leaders in every working unit.

STRUCTURE

Line Organization

This is the simplest structure, with direct emphasis on production, which may suit mass production for an undiscriminating market.

There is a direct line of control from the chairman, down through operational chiefs, to their managers and foremen. The relationships are direct and simple, but the control is autocratic, lacking flexibility, entirely dependent on judgement of the person at the top and tends to cramp initiative.

Line and Staff Organization

There is still an emphasis on production but, as specialist knowledge is increasingly required (e.g. accounting, market research, personnel, plant maintenance) certain advisory departments are set up, with their own functional heads and hierarchical systems.

This type of organization has some disadvantages. Line management are suspicious of 'specialists' when they see them as a threat to their executive functions. Specialist officers find faults, and may seek to take over some executive functions. There is a multiplicity of voices, there appears to be more than one boss, momentum is reduced by the need for more consultation and by difficult communications.

Recent Trends

The tendency for successful enterprises to grow in size, the increasing need for more specialist functions and the inefficient and unwieldy rigid line and staff concept have led to the development of decentralization. There has been the move to increasing local control, the delegation of decisions down the line, efficient coordination at each level, the recruitment of people with different training and backgrounds, and greater emphasis on management training.

The present-day manager needs to be quite a different person from the old concept of the autocratic boss. He still has to ensure the success and efficiency of his department, but he also has to lead a team of specialists in various fields, and ensure good informal and formal communications. He is the captain who must steer his ship successfully. This analogy is sometimes used to call this the 'ship system'.

The manager's task is increasingly complex with the development of industrial democracy, and the appointment of worker directors. He cannot rest on his authority alone, and he has to learn new techniques of leadership.

TRADE UNIONS

A trade union is any combination of persons having one or more of the following principal objects:

1. The regulation of relations between workmen and masters or between workmen and workmen or between masters and masters.
2. Imposing restrictive conditions on the conduct of any trade or business.
3. The provision of benefits to members.

Origin

Trade unions in the UK evolved in the latter part of the 17th century when the change in conditions of industry made it extremely unlikely for the skilled journeyman to become a master and when a sharp division occurred between capital and labour. It became necessary for the workmen to combine in order to maintain their standard of life.

In the beginning, trade unions were illegal, and even after the grant of some degree of legality in 1824 the law was still weighted heavily against them. It was possible for the law to be perverted as when, in 1834, six agricultural workers at Tolpuddle in Dorset were convicted of illegal oath taking at an initiation ceremony of the Grand National Consolidated Trade Union, and were deported to Australia.

Trade unions had to amend the law and prevent harmful interpretations of the law. A need for the trade unions to participate in the law-making process gave rise to the formation of the British Labour Party.

The trade unions had to organize the labour force in order to combat the harsh working conditions, the lack of health and safety measures, and the absence of financial assistance for the worker who was ill, injured or aged. The early efforts at organizing workmen were rendered very difficult by the severe class stratification of society and the fear that, should the workers get above their station, there would be terrible excesses as in revolutionary France. However, there were a number of enlightened people who saw the need for humanitarian measures, e.g. the industrialist Robert Owen and the aristocrat and politician, the Earl of Shaftesbury. Owen set up factories at New Lanark where the children received education, he refused to employ children under 10 years of age, he built improved houses with good sanitation and provided places for recreation. Shaftesbury was appalled by the fearful conditions of employment of young children and women. He was instrumental in the legislation forbidding the employment of women for underground labour in the mines, in appointing inspectors of mines, in limiting the hours of work of women and young persons, and in the Act instituting the 10 hours' limitation in textile factories. His humanitarianism arose from a deep religious conviction, and he thought that socialism and chartism were the two great demons in morals and politics. He was representative of the old land-owning class who were opposed to the rising industrialists.

Professionalism

In the latter half of the 19th century the larger unions set up headquarters in London with paid officials. With the growth of professionalism there came a wider and deeper interest in social reform.

Trade Union Congress

The first congress was held at Manchester in 1868, and it has met annually ever since. Executive duties are undertaken by the General Council which is organized to enter into discussions with the Government and the employer's bodies; for these purposes it has established certain specialist committees. It has taken the initiative on a number of reforms, e.g. the creation of the International Labour Office, universal secondary education, and the welfare state.

The centenary of the TUC, in 1968, was marked by the establishment of the TUC Institute of Occupational Health at the London School of Hygiene and Tropical Medicine.

The TUC Headquarters are at Congress House, Great Russell Street, London WC1. It provides a number of services to affiliated unions, not least in the role of mediator.

Types of Union

There are four broad types:

1. Craft Unions, the earliest type, which cover a single craft or group of craftsmen, e.g. Electrical Trades Union.

2. Industrial Unions, which cover all the workers in a particular industry or group of industries, e.g. Chemical Workers Union.

3. General Unions, which include especially general labourers, e.g. Transport and General Workers Union, National Union of General and Municipal Workers.

4. White-collar Unions; these have become more prominent as technical, scientific and service industries have grown in size.

Union Structure and Organization

The trade union is based on the local branch, sometimes called a Lodge or a Chapel. All members in the locality have the right to attend a branch meeting, they elect the officers and committee who deal with all union matters appropriate for local settlement. More important issues are referred to the district, regional or national office of the Union. The members also elect delegates to the Union's district and national committees and to the National Conference.

Trades Councils

These are permanent local bodies, first set up in the more important industrial towns in the middle of the 19th century. They are useful for the interchange of information and the discussion of purely local matters.

Shop Stewards

Originally the shop steward was appointed as a minor official of the union to inspect the membership cards and to recruit new members. As the union became bigger and the national office was more remote from the workplace, the shop steward became the focal point for local grievances and this tended to make him an aggressive agent, even a strike leader. During the First World War there were rapid changes in workshop practices, particularly in the engineering industry and there was replacement and dilution of much of the original labour force. The normal trade union officials could not cope with the increased pressures for negotiations in the workshops and the shop stewards' movement became very powerful, to the extent almost of devolving union power to the workshop as a step towards the workers' control of industry. The shop steward tended to rival the normal trade union leader. This was not to the liking of the leaders or the authorities, and a special committee was set up in 1916 under the chairmanship of J. H. Whitley to consider the problem.

Whitleyism

The Whitley Committee reported in 1917 and recommended:

1. The formation in the well-organized industries of joint industrial councils.

2. The appointment of works committees, representing equally the employers and workers.

3. Statutory regulation of wages in badly organized trades.

4. A permanent court of arbitration.

5. The Ministry of Labour to be authorized to hold enquiries regarding disputes.

In addition, the Committee advised the continuance of the present system whereby industry made their own agreements and settled their differences themselves.

Collective bargaining is applied to those arrangements under which wages and conditions of employment are settled by a bargain, in the form of an agreement made between employers or association of employers and workers' organizations. This bargain is usually reached by using the joint negotiating machinery which has evolved according to the varying needs and circumstances of the different trades and industries.

Joint Consultation

Many firms have arrangements for consultation between management and employees about matters of common concern which are outside the scope of the negotiating machinery; for example, changes or improvements in work methods and the safety, health and welfare of the employees. The passing of the Health and Safety at Work Act has provided a statutory requirement of consultative committees to study occupational health and safety.

Management and Unions

It is a mistake to think of trade union structure as a replica of company structure, with the officers and executive committee in the position of the chairman and board of directors, exerting authority which passes downwards to the individual member. It is more accurate to represent trade union organization as an inverted pyramid, with power residing in the shop-floor at the top and the elected officers at the bottom. It follows that it is futile for management to reach agreement with the elected officers if the shop-floor does not agree. Management's problem is to reach the individual worker and secure his understanding and support. This can no longer be done by the threat of the sack or the promise of additional financial incentives. It calls for a new type of management technique which, instead of enforcing obedience 'because I say so', is prepared to appeal to the intelligence and convince the worker that what is proposed is reasonable.

Trade Unionism in other Countries

The Industrial Revolution, with its need for trade unions, came early to Britain, and with the passage of time it became necessary for trade unionists to be politically active. In other countries the political activity came first, mainly as a result of the spread of socialist ideas, and the trade unions followed.

International Labour Organization

The TUC initiated the work which led to the creation of the ILO as an agency of the League of Nations in 1919. This organization is financed by member states and comprises one representative for each state, together with one representative of the workers and one for the employers. It has headquarters in Geneva and many branch offices throughout the world. The ILO is the only agency which survived the demise of the League of Nations and was carried forward into the present United Nations Organization.

THE INDUSTRIAL DOCTOR

In industry, the doctor has to fit into the organization and yet maintain his professional integrity and ethical standards. There are three ways in which this has been done:
1. The doctor as an independent expert.
2. The doctor as manager.
3. The doctor as company physician.

The Independent Expert

This has the advantage that an expert can be called in for a highly specialised matter. Provided his appointment is agreed jointly by the management and unions, or if he is the official Government expert, he will be seen to be entirely independent and his advice recognized to be unbiased. The disadvantage is that he will not have a detailed knowledge of the concern, and his advice may be limited to one or two special matters.

The Doctor in Management

One way of solving the dilemma of independence is to place the doctor squarely in the management hierarchy. Such appointments as Director, or Head, of Health and Safety are occurring. It is recognized that the doctor, with his long training and experience of human factors, is the right person to lead the team in health and safety. There are two possible important disadvantages:
   a. The doctor may need to spend time in 'managing', and less time on 'doctoring'.
   b. He is unequivocally a member of the management, however much he maintains his professional integrity.

The Doctor as Company Physician

This is a kind of half-way system in which the doctor is on the company payroll, yet he is accepted as an entirely independent adviser. He does not have any executive management function. However carefully he tries to maintain impartiality, from time to time he will be labelled as 'company lackey' or 'workers' friend' by one side or the other.
   This role requires constant vigilance, for human beings of every status can be very devious at times. The great advantage of this system is that the doctor has a detailed knowledge of the concern, and he can earn the respect of both

management and workers. Many doctors prefer this role to the other two alternatives.

Medical Ethics

Ethical rules for doctors practising occupational health are published by professional bodies (BMA, AMA, etc.). The following practical points add emphasis to these rules: The occupational health physician's role is to maintain health at work. Treatment, apart from first aid and immediate emergency measures, is not his principal function. This subject is discussed further in the chapter on the Practice of Occupational Medicine.

The employee has the right to know to what hazards he may be exposed at work. The doctor has a duty to inform the workers of these hazards, and of the results of medical examinations or special tests, and to present these results in a way which is readily and accurately understood.

Any medical report on a worker must not be made without that worker's knowledge, and his consent. Refusal to give consent may be overruled only in matters of statutory duty, public health, or factors involving the safety of others.

Medical judgement must not be influenced by conflicting interests.

All knowledge gained about individuals must be treated as confidential. Nothing of a confidential nature is to be disclosed without the patient's consent, whether to management, another doctor, or anyone else. The worker's personal physician understands the needs of his patient. The occupational health physician will see these needs, also the needs of his other patients — who are this worker's colleagues at work. One important task is to relate the patient's needs to the working group, and to interpret these within the resources of the organization. The occupational health doctor will have a good knowledge of the organization, he will often need to consult the general practitioner, who will have a good knowledge of the individual patient.

If it is necessary to examine a worker who is off sick, and therefore under active care of his general practitioner, that practitioner should be consulted first.

THE OCCUPATIONAL HEALTH NURSE

In the early days of industrial medicine some firms appointed nurses to assist in the works medical departments. They were appointed for their skill in treating the sick and injured. Some smaller firms found it practical to employ a nurse in place of training personnel for first aid duties. The nurse tended to be regarded as a sticker-on of plasters; her full professional ability was not used. In fact some managements took the view that it was good for the nurse to sit in her surgery and do her knitting, as this meant there were no injuries for her to treat. The nurse was restricted to the single role of treatment.

This attitude grossly undervalues and denigrates the ability of a professionally trained nurse. Taking an interest in the injuries she has to treat, she will make simple observations on the epidemiology of accidents, and she will be able to contribute to accident prevention. The nurse will then want to know about the materials and processes in her industry, and all the other factors involved with the prevention of disease and injury. The occupational health nurse now has a detailed post registration training in preventive nursing, and the syllabus for the Occupational Health Nursing Certificate will equip her for her work:

Health supervision at the place of work.

Health education.

Occupational safety.

Environmental monitoring.

Counselling.

The organization of an emergency treatment service for accident and illness at work.

Provision of a treatment service in certain situations.

Rehabilitation and resettlement.

Administration of the occupational health unit, including the development and maintenance of records.

Cooperation with outside agencies.

(For details and syllabus, see p. 21.)

There are not enough doctors to appoint one to every small industry, but many industries can appoint their own nurse. The fully trained occupational health nurse may well know more about the organization and hazards of her own factory than the doctor who can only spare an occasional visit. In a larger concern, the occupational health nurse is not a handmaiden to pass a sphygmomanometer to the doctor; she has her own valuable contribution to make in the occupational health team.

Many male nurses find that they have a successful and rewarding career in industry. This particularly applies to remote places of work, for example oil rigs, where it is not possible to have a doctor permanently on site, yet much more than ordinary first aid may be required. These medical auxiliaries have special training in traumatic surgery, medical emergencies, and resuscitation.

References

Harris, Cynthia J. (ed.) (1984) *Occupational Health Nursing Practice*. Bristol, Wright.

Pemberton, Doreen (1965) *Essentials of Occupational Health Nursing*. London, Arlington Books.

Tyrer F. H. (1961) *Occupational Health Nursing*. London, Ballière Tindall & Cox.

Formerly there were two means by which industrial accidents were notified. These were based on different criteria, they produced different data and led to some confusion. A reportable accident was one where the consequent injury caused an absence from work of three days or more. These were reported to the factory inspectorate. A recorded accident was one where the injury was recorded for insurance purposes, under the National Insurance (Industrial Injuries) Act.

The Notification of Accidents and Dangerous Occurrences Regulations 1980 seeks to rationalise reporting procedure.

DEFINITIONS

An accident is an unexpected, unexplained occurrence which may involve injury (ILO).

The regulations define four types of incident:

i. Fatal accident
ii. Major injury accident
iii. Other accidents
iv. Dangerous occurrences

Fatal accidents have to be reported if they arise out of or in connection with work whether the person who dies is employed or not.

An accident resulting in a major injury which arises out of or in connection with work has to be reported. A major injury is defined as:

a. Fracture of the skull, spine, or pelvis;
b. Fracture of any bone
   i. In the arm, other than a bone in the wrist or hand;
   ii. In the leg, other than a bone in the ankle or foot;
c. Amputation of a hand or foot,
d. The loss of sight of an eye; or
e. Any other injury which results in the person injured being admitted into hospital as an in-patient for more than 24 hours, unless that person is detained only for observation.

In this type of case there is no need to assess the degree of incapacity for work or resulting disability. The fact that an accident has occurred and the person has sustained one of the injuries listed above means that it must be reported. If the extent of the injury is not apparent at the time of the accident or if the injured person has not been admitted to hospital immediately it is still counted as a major accident if one of those injuries is confirmed or more than 24 hours is spent in hospital other than for observation.

Fatal and major injury accidents must immediately be reported to the Health and Safety Executive.

Other accidents resulting in injury are not reported to the Health and Safety Executive. All such injuries in occupations now covered by the Health and Safety at Work Act will be recorded for national insurance purposes. Employees have a duty to report accidents which result in personal injury. Usually an entry is required on Form BI 510. If the employee makes a claim for Industrial Injury Benefit the employer has to make a report to the Department of Health and Social Security. Information through these sources will be passed by that Department to the Health and Safety Executive. No direct reporting by the employer to the Health and Safety Executive is required.

Dangerous occurrences are events which, although not necessarily causing injury, have the potential for doing so, e.g. explosure of a pressure vessel, collapse of a crane. A full definition of dangerous occurrences is given in Appendix 1, Schedule 1, Part 1 of the Health and Safety series booklet HS(R)5 *The Notification of Accidents and Dangerous Occurrences*.

ACCIDENT STATISTICS

It is difficult to find a satisfactory criterion which can easily be applied to separate trivial from serious injuries. In one study of two similar factories, the ratio between 'severe' (reportable) and 'minor' (non-reportable but recorded) accidents differed from 1 : 20 to 1 : 500.

To avoid including the large and very variable numbers of all trivial injuries, accident statistics are usually based on Reportable Accident data.

It is acknowledged that there are many factors which determine whether a worker will find it necessary to absent himself after injury, including: morale, the type of work, and the employer's ability to provide immediate treatment and rehabilitation. Therefore caution must be used when comparing data.

Frequency Rate

$$FR = \frac{E}{C} \times 100\ 000.$$

Severity Rate

$$SR = \frac{F}{C} \times 100\ 000.$$

E = Number of accidents causing a loss of working time in a given period.
C = Total man hours worked in a given period.
F = Total hours lost through accidents occurring in a given period.

If it is difficult to calculate the total number of man hours worked, the incident rate can be used.

Incident Rate

$$IR = \frac{E}{N} \times 1000.$$

Where N = the average number of persons employed during the given period.

Fatal Accidents

Rate per 1000 men at risk

Deep sea fishing	1·4
Coal mining	0·4
Construction industry	0·2
Manufacturing industry	0·04

Fatal accidents in offices. The rate per 1000 at risk is not available but the total figures for the UK in 1975 compare as follows:

Premises covered by the:

	Fatal accidents
Factories Act	427
Offices, Shops and Railway Premises Act	16
Mines and Quarries Act	81
Agriculture (Health and Safety) Act	34
(Health and Safety Executive Statistics)	

Types of Accidents

Although some industries have particular risks, the overall pattern shows that machinery is not the major cause of accidents.

Percentage of all industrial accidents, UK, 1968

Handling 27·1	Transport 8·2
Machinery 17·5	Struck by falling objects 7·2
Persons falling 14·7	Hand tools 7
Striking against objects 9·0	Others 9·3

ACCIDENT PREVENTION

Man is fallible and machinery can go wrong; it is better to recognize the inevitability of these weaknesses and attack them than to regard accidents as inexplicable arrangements of fate.

Education

As the machinery and equipment are to be used or operated by man, engineers should have some basic training in anatomy, physiology, toxicology and ergonomics.

Safe working is part of the skill and should be learnt with other skills. It should be taught at school before the apprentice, trainee or operative enters industry.

Human Factors

Certain tasks may need certain abilities or standards of fitness, and appropriate medical selection is needed.

Safety performance will be improved by training and job experience. It will be impaired by fatigue, illness and alcoholism.

Accident proneness varies between individuals and seems to be a temporary phenomenon. Some workers have described the results of tests of personality traits and have related these to accident proneness; validation is difficult.

Shift work seems to have variable effects. In purely manual tasks, there are less accidents on the night shift, but this may be partly due to the different working conditions prevailing at night, the slower working pace, greater freedom of movement, and diminished danger from transport. In tasks which are not entirely manual, some surveys have shown that more errors occur in the hours shortly following midnight.

The effect of age is difficult to assess; the young are more agile but are inexperienced, job experience increases with age. The severity of accidents, and the resulting degree of disability tend to increase among older workers.

Environmental Factors

If man has to learn and perform certain tasks, his resources of adaptation should not be stressed by an unfavourable environment.

In 1922 Vernon showed that in a group of munition workers, the accident rate was least when the temperature was 19·5°C (67°F). There was a 40 per cent increase in the accident rate when the temperature was raised by 5°C (10°F).

Ventilation, lighting, working posture, instrument displays, communications, rest and meal breaks should all be designed to reduce fatigue. Good conditions will improve productivity as well as safety.

Management Aspects

In the early stages of the Industrial Revolution labour was cheap and expendable. The deplorable injuries and loss of life are no longer acceptable, both for humane and economic reasons. Unfortunately, even now good accident prevention measures are sometimes declared to be too costly, and there is an apparent conflict between safety and productivity. This conflict has not been the sole preserve of management, for sometimes workers have sought 'danger money' rather than safe working.

One important factor in changing attitudes is the direct involvement of the worker through worker safety representatives.

Management should publish a *safety policy* which sets out the firm's commitment to safety, and make financial provisions for carrying out the policy. Management and worker representatives should set an example by always obeying safety rules, e.g. the use of safety equipment and clothing. *Safety officers* may be appointed to advise, inspect and instruct, though there is a danger if any responsibility for safety is removed from line management. Line managers as well as operatives should receive appropriate *safety training*. Hazardous tasks should be identified and suitable *codes of practice* designed.

Employees' *job descriptions* should include a safety and health element.

Productivity and other *bonus* or *incentive* schemes should be designed to include and improve safety factors. *Employee participation* can be improved by *hazard reporting* schemes and by *joint consultation*.

FIRST AID

The Health and Safety (First Aid) Regulations 1981 came into operation on 1 July 1982, accompanied by a Code of Practice. Their scope is more comprehensive than previous Regulations in that they apply to *all* places of employment and to the self-employed; but there is also a degree of flexibility which takes into account the wide variation in hazards, work and location.

The employer is required to provide adequate first aid facilities and suitably trained people to supervise them.

Suitable Persons. Three categories are recognized:

1. First Aider — holding a current First Aid certificate approved by the Health and Safety Executive.

2. Occupational First Aider — holding a current Occupational First Aid certificate approved by the Health and Safety Executive (usually with additional training in hazards specific to the establishment).

3. Appointed Persons — who will take charge, call the ambulance and generally organize the action to be taken for serious illness or injury. (Not acceptable as full-time alternatives to First Aiders unless number of employees small and hazards low.)

Numbers Required

1. Low hazard establishments (shops, offices, banks)
   Less than 150 employees — Appointed Person.
   More than 150 employees — 1 First Aider per 150 employees.
2. Greater hazards (factories, warehouses, etc.)
   Less than 50 employees — Appointed person.
   More than 50 employees — First Aider
   More than 150 employees — 1 First Aider per 150 employees.
3. Unusual hazards (some chemical companies, shipbuilding, etc.)
   The above numbers may need to be increased.

If employees of more than one firm are working on the same site, e.g. construction sites, contractors working in factories, first aid facilities may be shared. Agreements to this effect should be in writing, and all employees should be informed of the arrangement.

Training

1. Any organization may train first aiders and occupational first aiders provided the syllabus and trainers are approved by the Health and Safety Executive.

2. There must be examinations by independent examiners, at least one of whom must be a doctor or nurse with experience of first aid at work. The examination must include resuscitation, the control of bleeding and the management of the unconscious patient.

3. Certificates are valid for 3 years. Before recertification candidates must have attended a refresher course lasting at least one day.

4. The course and examination must last at least 4 days, and must include:
resuscitation, control of bleeding, treatment of shock
treatment of the unconscious patient
dressing and immobilization of injured parts
contents of first aid boxes
transport of the sick and injured
treatment of injuries, burns and scalds
simple record keeping
poisons
personal hygiene
communication and delegation in emergency.

For occupational first aiders, the course must, in addition, include:
safety and hygiene
keeping of detailed records
hazards specific to the undertaking, e.g. chemical.

Instructors. Must be:
Doctors or nurses with knowledge of first aid.
Graduate lecturers or qualified teachers with a current first aid certificate.
Lay instructors with a certificate from an approved organization.
First aiders and occupational first aiders may apply to become instructors. The St. John and St. Andrews organizations and the British Red Cross Society have revised their training syllabus, and now require *all* instructors to have attended an instructors' course and obtained a certificate.

First Aid Boxes (Recommended marking white cross on green.) Must be clearly identified and contain

| Item | Numbers of employees | | | | |
	1–5	6–10	11–50	51–100	101–150
Guidance card	1	1	1	1	1
Individually wrapped sterile adhesive dressings	10	20	40	40	60
Sterile eye pads, with attachment	1	2	4	6	8
Triangular bandages	1	2	4	6	8
Sterile coverings for serious wounds (where applicable)	1	2	4	6	8
Safety pins	6	6	12	12	12
Medium-sized sterile unmedicated dressings	3	6	8	10	12
Large sterile unmedicated dressings	1	2	4	6	10
Extra large sterile unmedicated dressings	1	2	4	6	8

Where sterile water or sterile normal saline in disposable containers needs to be kept near the first-aid box because tap water is not available, at least the following quantities should be kept:

	Number of employees			
	1–10	11–50	51–100	101–150
Sterile water or saline in disposable containers (where tap water is not available)	1	3	6	6

These boxes should be provided at places where the first aid room cannot be reached in three minutes. In certain cases other regulations such as the Hydrogen Cyanide (fumigation of buildings) Regulations and the Food Hygiene (general) Regulations specify certain other items. These should be kept in first aid boxes or similar containers, in addition to the items listed above.

First Aid Room. Recommended for establishments with more than 400 employees, or less than this in special circumstances. If not constantly manned, should have first aider nearby or on call. Room should be readily available, not used for any other purpose and give easy access to transport. It should be ventilated, heated, lit, maintained and cleaned daily with removal of all refuse. It should be large enough to hold a couch and allow people to move about. The door should be large enough to admit a stretcher or wheelchair. There should be a waiting-room with chairs. The room should be identified and have a sign outside giving the names and location of first aiders. There should be a telephone or other means of communication, and it should preferably be near toilets.

The room should contain:
sink with hot and cold water
drinking water
paper towels
soap and nail brush
smooth top working surface
sterile dressings
thermometers
couch, pillow and blankets
a store
clean garments
refuse container

Self-employed. Are advised to provide themselves with a small travelling first aid kit.

All employees should be informed of the location of first aid material and personnel, and kept informed of changes.

The Regulations do not apply to diving operations, merchant shipping, vessels registered outside UK, mines and Armed Forces.

Previous Regulations Repealed
Agriculture (Safety, Health & Welfare Provisions) Act, Secs. 6(1) and (4).
Factories Act, 1961. Sec. 61.
Offices Shops & Railway Premises Act, Sec. 24.
First Aid Boxes (Miscellaneous Industries) First Aid Order.

Bibliography

Human Factors and Safety. CIS Information Sheet No. 15 Geneva, International Labour Office.

Chapter 6 Rehabilitation

Definition

In general sense, means restoration of maximum possible *function* after illness or injury.

Industrial rehabilitation means restoration of maximum possible *earning capacity*.

Basic Principle

Work at optimum point in recovery is therapeutic. Just as in every illness and injury (other than minor) there is a period during which rest from work is an essential part of treatment, so there is a point at which *suitable work* becomes an essential part of treatment. Beyond this, continued idleness is positively harmful, and will lead to incomplete recovery of function, perhaps actual deterioration, together with erosion of morale and will to work.

Hence identification of optimum point for starting some form of work is crucial.

This depends on clinical judgement in every case. Normally it is the point at which:

1. Traditional therapy, e.g. physiotherapy and medication, appears to have achieved all the improvement possible.

2. The general condition is such that regular attendance at some place of work is possible.

Who determines this point? Normally the GP or consultant responsible for treatment in the early stages of illness or injury.

What happens next?

If the patient is still retained on the books of an employer, this is the time to establish contact with the employer to decide, first, whether he is fit for his previous work, and if not, what alternative work within his present capacity can be offered. Where there is a works medical officer, this is probably best done through him. Failing this, the Employment Medical Adviser will undertake the necessary investigation of the possibilities, if asked; or in a few cases, especially with smaller firms, direct contact between GP or consultant and management may be possible, and more appropriate.

Communication

Communication must be established *early*. The communications gulf normally existing between doctors carrying out treatment and industrial managements is the biggest obstacle to successful rehabilitation, and the patient's interests require that it should be bridged.

Many managements are more than willing to modify or change an employee's work for a while if this is in the interests of his rehabilitation, particularly if he has been the victim of a works accident or is a long-service employee. But without specific guidance as to the necessary restrictions they are afraid of doing him harm. The doctor for his part may have a very unclear idea of the working conditions and the range and requirements of alternative work, so tends to play for safety by prolonging the period of certified incapacity.

Successful rehabilitation therefore depends on communication.

Role of Employers

Some large employers, e.g. Vauxhall Motors, British Leyland, run special rehabilitation workshops providing suitably graded work for their own sick and injured employees.

Resettlement with the original employer is usually the ideal to be aimed at, if it is feasible.

Government Agencies

If the patient has lost his previous employment the help of the Disablement Resettlement Officer should be sought. These officers are attached to District Offices of the Manpower Services Commission, which also runs the Jobcentres which have replaced the old Employment Exchanges. (In a few localities there are DROs based on hospitals.)

Broadly, their function is to advise and assist in all employment problems of disabled people. They handle applications for placing on the Disabled Persons' Register (q.v.), make arrangements for admission to Government (or other) Rehabilitation Centres, and help disabled people whose capacity for work has been assessed to find suitable work or obtain vocational training. They are able to call on the Employment Medical Advisory Service for assessment of the significance of disabilities in relation to work. Their clients may be referred by a doctor or social worker, or seek their help spontaneously.

Ideally, the DRO's help should be sought in the early stages of illness or disability, so as to reduce the inevitable time-lags which are an impediment to successful rehabilitation. It is often not appreciated that it is not necessary to wait until a doctor has certified a patient fit for work before any approach is made. All too often, months are allowed to elapse after partial recovery before the first approach is made. It is for this reason that the experiment has been tried in a few selected hospitals of basing the DRO there, so that consultants are aware of his existence and functions, and he is aware at an early date of patients likely to need his services.

REHABILITATION CENTRES

There are 27 Employment Rehabilitation Centres (formerly known as Industrial Rehabilitation Units) in Great Britain. Their aims are twofold:

1. To re-establish a pattern of regular hours of work and rebuild confidence and morale; and

2. To assess individual fitness for future employment, or in appropriate cases, for vocational training.

Case conferences attended by medical officer, occupational psychologist, chief instructor, social worker, rehabilitation officer and manager are held on intake before discharge.

A minority of those passing through ERCs who show potential and motivation for training in specific skills and crafts are referred either to Government Training Centres or receive grants for training in technical colleges and similar institutions. Others may return to their original employment, and it is the task of the DRO to seek to place the remainder in jobs of the type considered suitable by the Centre.

There are, in addition to Government Rehabilitation Centres, a number of voluntary institutions partly supported by public funds, such as St Loye's College at Exeter and Queen Elizabeth College, Leatherhead, which are residential, and where assessment, rehabilitation and training form part of a continuous process, which is the ideal. Their results tend to be better, partly for this reason but also because they are highly selective in their choice of applicants.

REMPLOY

Remploy is a Government corporation operating 94 factories in Great Britain, set up specifically to provide jobs for disabled persons. It operates on a normal commercial basis, although receiving an annual subvention.

SHELTERED WORKSHOPS AND SHELTERED INDUSTRIAL GROUPS

Most of these are operated by local authorities, and are designed for those people whose physical or mental handicap is so severe that they are unable to obtain or retain jobs on the open labour market. Most of the work consists of simple jobs contracted out by local industries — manual assembly of small components, wrapping and packaging of small goods for retail sale, and the like. The Industrial Therapy Organization in Bristol provides similar workshops, which employ large numbers of patients from local mental hospitals. Voluntary bodies such as the Spastics Society also provide them.

Sheltered industrial groups, formerly known as enclaves, are small groups of severely disabled people working under special supervision in ordinary and undifferentiated working conditions alongside able-bodied people.

They were first established in 1960 and are recognized as an additional and especially cost effective way of providing sheltered employment for severely disabled people. Although most of the early groups were established in parks and gardens schemes, many have now been settled in other working environments, for example, kitchens, laundries, industrial premises and commercial undertakings.

Their aim is to provide severely disabled people with the opportunity of doing a normal job, earning a normal wage in a normal working environment.

The Disabled Persons (Employment) Acts 1944 and 1958

Government Rehabilitation Centres were set up under this legislation and Disablement Resettlement Officers appointed, under the direction of the then Ministry of Labour (now Manpower Services Commission).

Essential provisions are:

1. Maintenance of a Disabled Persons' Register. Registration is voluntary, and the DRO can accept an applicant for registration if the disability is obvious, e.g. loss of a limb, confinement to a wheelchair. Otherwise medical evidence is required to the effect that there is a disability which is liable to cause a substantial impairment of the individual's prospects of obtaining or retaining employment.

2. Requirement on all employers of 20 or more people to include a quota (which has remain unchanged at 3%) of Registered Disabled Persons in their work force.

Sanctions on employers falling below the quota are relatively mild. Until it is filled, local Jobcentres will refer only registered disabled for any vacancies which occur. Most employers have no difficulty in complying with or exceeding the quota by encouraging existing employees with minor disabilities to apply for registration, so that on the whole the Act has not helped the unemployed disabled to the extent that its sponsors probably intended. The quota system has recently been under review and its abolition considered, on the grounds that:

1. There are probably at least as many non-registered as registered disabled persons.

2. It has been calculated that if every employer were in fact employing his 3 % quota, the numbers on the Register would be insufficient to enable the requirement to be met. In other words, the requirement is only spasmodically enforced, and there are now a great many well-disposed employers who are employing considerably more than their quota.

The rehabilitation, placement and training facilities of Government agencies are equally available to registered and non-registered disabled people.

Chapter 7 Ergonomics

Definition

The application of the human biological sciences in conjunction with engineering sciences to achieve the optimum mutual adjustment of man and his work, the benefits being measured in terms of human efficiency and well-being.

Scope

Ergonomics may apply anatomy, physiology, biomechanics, ergometrics, psychology and cybernetics. In North America the term 'human engineering' is used to mean the design of the machine or work environment to suit the human operator.

Posture

1. Standing. Work is often done standing because no thought has been given to allowing the operator to sit down. If work must be done standing:

There must be sufficient foot and knee room for mobility and balance.

The worker should not need to adopt a bent posture.

The working height should be such as to allow the use of the arm muscles to the best mechanical advantage.

Bench working height is usually 100–115 cm.

Posture will be difficult to maintain, and will lead to overactivity and fatigue of postural muscles when there is a small standing platform restricting changes of stance, the trunk has to be flexed to reach over the work and one foot has to be used to operate a control.

2. Sitting

Seat height should be such that the feet can be placed firmly on the floor, or on a foot rest. The knees are at a right angle. The seat should not compress the calf or back of the thighs.

The *working surface* should allow space underneath for the legs to be moved, and crossed if wanted. The arms should work with the forearms near horizontal; therefore typists' desks usually have a lower working surface than clerk's desks.

The *back rest* should support the lumbar region.

Adjustable seats will allow for maximum comfort, but fixed seats, properly designed, will suit about 80% of people. The usual dimensions are:

Height of seat 43 cm (range 42–50 cm).

Height of worktop 67–70 cm.

Seat depth 38 cm.
Seat width 40 cm, wider if arm rests are fitted.
In the sitting position there is less postural strain, but also less mobility. The work should be within normal arm's reach. If work has to be reached for, it is better to have the seat on wheels, a slide or a pivot.

Repeated Movements

Tools and machinery should be designed to give the best mechanical advantage to the limbs which operate them, to use the muscles most effectively and prevent fatigue. The design of a screwdriver handle is a good example; an ovoid knob will fit comfortably in the palm, a wider diameter will allow an easier grip and better leverage. Repeated strain on particular muscle groups can cause occupational cramps or occupational tenosynovitis.

Lifting and Carrying

The handling of objects is the most frequent cause of industrial accidents, and back injuries account for a large proportion of sickness absence. Wherever possible mechanical means should be used for lifting and moving heavy objects. Where this is impracticable, the operator should be trained in the correct method of lifting and the work should be so designed that this method can be used.

It should be possible for the operator to obtain a good hand hold, using the whole palm of the hand. He should have sufficient space to keep his feet apart, to provide a good balance, and he should not have to twist his body whilst lifting or carrying. The arms should be held close to the sides and fully extended, the back should be kept straight and the body raised by extending the bent legs. Loads should not have to be lifted above shoulder height.

It is difficult to define a maximum load which should be lifted. In various Regulations under the Factories Act different maximum weights have been prescribed. In general, if the load approaches or exceeds 50% of the individual's body weight it is likely to cause strain or loss of balance.

The International Labour Conference adopted the Maximum Weight Recommendation which states that 'where the maximum permissible weight which may be transported manually by one adult worker is more than 55 kg, measures should be taken as speedily as possible to reduce it to that level'. This weight is a suggested upper limit and applies to ideal conditions. It is suggested that the maximum weight for women should be about 50% of that for adult male workers.

Ergometrics

The static medical examination gives little indication of the individual's ability to perform heavy physical work. Extreme physical demands may be placed upon workers in certain tasks, e.g. in extremes of heat and exertion when repairing brick furnaces, in mines rescue teams, and in firefighters.

Some measure of physical working capacity can be obtained by measuring maximum oxygen consumption during exercise. This can be determined indirectly by measuring the heart rate response to exercise tests, usually (as in the Harvard step test) by measuring the heart rate recovery after measured exercise.

THE THERMAL ENVIRONMENT

Thermal Comfort

Thermal comfort depends on: Temperature (ambient temperature and heat from radiation); Humidity; Air movement.

Measuring the Thermal Environment

Temperature: by dry bulb thermometer.
Radiant heat: globe thermometer; the bulb is in a 6-in copper globe, painted matt black. If there is over −7°C (20°F) difference between the globe and dry bulb thermometer, normal air movement will not be sufficient in reducing heat gain by radiation.
Humidity: Measured by the difference between wet and dry bulb thermometers. A whirling hygrometer (sling psychrometer) holding both wet and dry bulbs is whirled round to give a reasonably constant air flow over the bulbs. Relative humidity is read off the chart supplied with the instrument.
Air movement: (i) by Kata thermometer: an alcohol thermometer with a large bulb. It is heated by immersing in hot water, dried, and the rate of cooling measured. Velocity of air movement can be read off from accompanying tables. There are three ranges of thermometer; (ii) for measuring high velocities, especially directional air flow and draughts, a velometer (swing vane instrument) is used. Its lower limit is about 40 ft per minute.

Effective Temperature

An index giving a measure of the warmth of the environment, combining temperature, humidity and air movement. It is referred to the standard conditions of still and saturated air, so that the effective temperature of an environment indicates the temperature of still air, saturated with water vapour, in which an equivalent sensation of warmth was experienced by the subjects in a long series of tests. Its main disadvantage is that it makes no allowance for radiant heat.

Equivalent Temperature

This is a scale of warmth sometimes used by heating and ventilating engineers. It takes into account radiation, air temperature and air movement, but it makes no allowance for humidity.

Corrected Effective Temperature

This is similar to the effective temperature, but it includes radiant heat.

Ideal Conditions for Comfort

Temperature about 65°F (18·5°C).
Air movement 1–2 ft per second.
Relative humidity over 60%, less than 70%.
Temperature at floor higher than at head level.

Statutory Standards

1. Space. Factories Act and Offices and Shops Act: Space for every person employed shall not be less than 400 ft^3.

2. Confined Space. Factories Act, Section 30, controls working inside confined spaces in which dangerous fumes are likely to be present. Size of egress not less than 18 in × 16 in. Suitable breathing apparatus must be worn, or else the space must be certified by a responsible person as safe to enter without it. Belts and ropes for rescue, and breathing apparatus must be examined monthly, and the signed reports kept for inspection. Some of those working in a confined space must be trained in methods of restoring respiration.

3. Ventilation. The Factories Act and the Offices and Shops Act both require the provision of adequate supplies of fresh or artificially purified air but no firm standards are laid down.

4. Temperature. The Factories Act requires a minimum temperature one hour after the start of work of 15·5°C (60°F) where a substantial proportion of the work is carried out sitting. Thermometers must be displayed. Requirements of the Offices and Shops Act are similar, but the temperature should be 16°C (60·8°F).

5. Humidity. The Factories Act requires an occupier to give notice to the Inspectorate if he intends to use artificial humidity. There must be no artificial humidification if the wet bulb exceeds 22·5°C (72·5°F) (in certain processes 26·6°C (80°F)), and there must usually be at least 2·2°C (4°F) difference.

Body Heat Production and Loss

The heat generated through metabolism must be dissipated to the environment. Metabolic heat generation is greatly influenced by the activity level of the individual, varying between 1·8 kcal/min for office work to 7 kcal/min for heavy manual work. The heat generated by the body is dissipated to the environment by radiation, convection and evaporation. Radiation and convection cease to be effective above 35°C (95°F); the heat loss is then entirely by the evaporation of sweat.

At rest, under comfortable conditions, about 10% of the body's maximum evaporative capacity will be used. Between 10 and 25% will still be comfortable, between 25 and 70% will be tolerable, but over 70% will be extremely uncomfortable. In a hot mine, in one shift, a man may lose 8 kg of sweat, containing 20 g of salt. The amount of salt in the sweat is reduced by acclimatization. The high loss of salt in excessive sweating will have to be replaced to avoid chloride depletion.

Protection

Workers in hot conditions can be protected by:

Facilitation of cooling by providing air movement.

Providing screens to protect against radiant heat.

Providing frequent moderate drinks of water, containing salt.

Frequent rest periods.

Regular temperature recordings in severe heat stress.

Heat-protective clothing.

In moderate heat the worker may wear as little as possible, in order to facilitate evaporation of the sweat. In hotter conditions he may need special protective clothing with thick layers to protect against heat radiation and an outer aluminized surface to reflect the heat. In even hotter conditions a piped air supply can be provided underneath the porous clothing, to provide for improved evaporation of sweat and a reversed temperature gradient through the clothing.

Vision

The visual functions which are commonly tested are:

Acuity: the requirements vary according to the task.

Field: important in transport.

Colour vision: of little importance, except where colour coding may be used and usually a practical test is given. Little relevance in transport as traffic signals can usually be safely read, a special signal test can be conducted if necessary.

Binocular vision: important in some industries, e.g. transport, also there may be reason to exclude people with monocular vision from tasks which have a serious eye hazard.

Stereoscopic vision and depth perception: important in some tasks, e.g. crane drivers. Beware of vision-testing apparatus, as the driver may adapt by using other mechanisms for determining distance. A practical test is usually better and more acceptable than an instrument test.

Factors Involved in Seeing

1. Size of object. Not its physical size, but the angle subtended at the eye. It may be necessary to adopt standards of near or distance vision.

2. Illumination. Ability to perceive fine detail increases with luminance. Within the limits of comfort; the greater the illumination, the smaller the pupil, the greater the depth of focus and the less strain on the eye.

3. Contrast. When contrast between objects is poor, discrimination is improved by increasing illumination.

4. Movement. Speed of perception is increased as illumination increases.

5. Glare. When the background is brighter than the object to be observed, it will impair visual acuity.

Vision Standards. In certain tasks standards of vision are required, for example: Public Service Vehicle and Heavy Goods Vehicle driving: the corrected visual acuity must not be worse than 6/9 in one eye and 6/12 in the other eye, with full visual fields and not less than 6/60 uncorrected in both eyes. Good standards of vision are required on recruitment for the Police Force, where high speed driving and traffic patrol duties are involved, unaided acuity of at least 6/6 in one eye and

6/12 in the other. In the Fire Service, where the fireman cannot wear glasses with breathing apparatus, unaided visual acuity of at least 6/12 in each eye is required.

Units of Lighting

The *lumen* (luminous flux) is the quantity of light emitted by a light source.

The *candela* (luminous intensity) is a luminous flux emitted per unit of solid angle in a given direction.

The *lux* (illumination) is the luminous flux that strikes a unit of area. 1 lux = 1 lumen/m^2.

The *candela/m^2* (luminance or brightness) is the luminous flux reflected by a surface.

Contrast is the relative luminance between an object and its background.

The *glare index* is a calculation based on various measurements of light distribution reflection from surfaces and room dimensions. There is a limiting glare index recommended for various tasks to be found in the Illuminating Engineering Society Code.

Levels of Illumination. Some Regulations were made under the Factories Act during the Second World War (Standards of Lighting Regulations 1941). These Regulations prescribe a minimum of 0·5 foot-candles for passageways, 2 foot-candles for general illumination, and 6 foot-candles where work is actually being done. (1 foot-candle = 10 lux.) These standards are out of date, and there are a number of recommended levels; the following is a representative selection:

Work	*Lux*
Canteens, cloakrooms, corridors, stairs	100–150
Engine assembly work	300
Office work	400–800
Fine assembly, e.g. precision instruments	1 500
Watch making	3 000

Information Displays. Many tasks in modern industry require the reading of displays of instruments. The following factors are important:

1. Quick reading. Digital presentation is best for giving rapid information (it obviates parallax). A pointer dial indicates change more readily.

2. Accuracy. The instrument should be capable of being read accurately, but not with more accuracy than is necessary.

The display should not be subject to reading errors or incorrect interpretation. The information should be instantly available in the desired form; it should not be necessary for the observer to convert to different units.

Unnecessary information should not be displayed.

AUTOMATION

Definition

The use of machines to run machines. In full automation man has only to design the equipment, and with the evolution of computers and miniaturized electronic equipment the final step of removing man from the process is possible. However, in most automated processes man is still needed to exercise overall control and to make decisions which are outside the competence of the equipment.

The Worker in Automation

There are both advantages and disadvantages to the worker:

Advantages. There is less bother with the minutiae of production, giving the worker more time to control and supervise.

Automated processes are easy to enclose totally.

There is less close supervision and less handling, the worker is removed from dangerous materials or processes.

Automation improves the workers' environment.

Disadvantages. There is less physical work to do, so physical fitness may deteriorate.

There will be a reduction in the manpower required by industry, the monotonous and routine jobs being lost first, and eventually some craftsmen will find their skills are unnecessary.

Watching displays or standing by for an alarm will create boredom.

The speeding up and enlargement of the process will give the worker much greater responsibility; a wrong decision could be disastrous.

The worker is removed from the process and there is less intimate involvement with the work.

The worker will tend to become isolated and lonely.

Work design

The above factors should be considered in job design. When man is placed in a man–machine system he should not be expected to adapt totally to the machine – the system should be designed to use man's contribution efficiently. If there is too little for him to do there will be boredom, if there is too much he will make mistakes. In systems where an operator has to intervene only when there is an alarm he should be kept alerted by some deliberate intervention during the shift, even by introducing some deliberate false alarms.

HOURS OF WORK

In the early days of the Industrial Revolution the novel and expensive machinery was worked for as long as possible, and people commonly worked 14 hours a day; even young children were employed for long hours. In the early part of the 19th century a working day of 12 hours was usual. The following rules are quoted from the Rules and Regulations to be observed by workmen at Robert Stephenson's Locomotive Works, in 1838:

> The Bell will be rung at 6 o'clock in the Morning, at 6 o'clock in the Evening throughout the Year for a Days' Work, except during the Months of November, December and January, when work will commence at 7

o'clock in the Morning, and close at 6 o'clock; and on Saturdays the Day's Work will end at 4 o'clock.

Any Workman washing himself, putting on his Coat, or making any other preparation for leaving Work before the Bell rings, to be fined.... 1s 0d.

By the early part of the 20th century the 48-hour week was common. The demands on industry, especially in munitions manufacture, during the First World War prompted long working hours, but it was shown that excessive hours of work had an adverse effect on production.

Since 1919 the International Labour Conference has adopted a number of recommendations, notably the standard 48-hour week with a 8- or 9-hour day, and in 1962 the progressive attainment of the 40-hour week.

There should be a main meal break during the day, and it is usual to have a number of short breaks, according to the type of work being done. Tasks requiring a high degree of concentration or of physical effort are usually performed more effectively when there are some short rest pauses.

Women and Young Persons

Women and young persons (under the age of 18) are protected from long hours and from night work. Section 86 of the Factories Act makes the following provisions:

The total hours worked must not exceed 9 in any day or 48 in any week.

The period of employment must not exceed 11 hours in any day and must not begin earlier than 7.00 a.m. or end later than 8.00 p.m. (1.00 p.m. on Saturdays).

There must be an interval of at least half an hour after every 4½ hour work period.

If an interval of not less than 10 minutes is allowed during the work period, that period may be increased to 5 hours.

Section 97 of the Factories Act allows the occupier to apply for authorization to employ women and young persons on shift work, but work at nights and on Sundays is still forbidden. There are a few limited exceptions affecting work in launderies and in certain food processes.

This legislation in the UK, which has a historical background, has certain anomalies. The law protects women in factories, but not in other forms of employment. For example, a nurse in a busy surgical ward may work very strenuously for a 12-hour night shift. With increasing interest in womens' rights, the Equal Opportunities Commission is investigating these anomalies. The legislation, which was designed to protect women, is seen as restrictive to them, barring them from some of the more highly remunerative jobs and restricting their prospects for promotion.

Shift Work

Work covering the whole 24-hour period may be necessary in industry where the production process cannot be halted. It is also demanded in certain service industries, e.g. police, fire, medical services. The day may be divided into two 12-hour shifts, or more commonly three 8-hour shifts.

Biological Aspects. Apart from the night predators, most animals sleep at night. Sleep is not the only biological function to show this rhythm; body temperature, pulse rate, blood pressure, renal excretion and endocrine activity all show a 24-hour rhythm (Circadian rhythm). These rhythmic changes keep their constant periodicity even when man is kept in total darkness for several months.

When the diurnal rhythm is artificially changed some slow adaptation will occur. The slower the change, the easier the adaptation. Rapid time changes in transcontinental travel, crossing time zones, produces a fatigue (jet lag) which was not observed when journeys were made by ship.

Shift Systems. Adaptation to reversal of activity (work at night, sleep by day) is never complete. For this, and for social reasons, some form of alternating shift system is usually preferred. There are two main types; a weekly change, or a short (one- or two-day) change.

Arguments in favour of both have been made, in the two-day change there is no time for any adaptation, and the normal rhythm is easily restored on rest days and holidays. It can be argued that this is less harmful than breaking a partial adaptation that may have occurred after 7 days on the same shift time.

A study of workers in one factory where the shift was changed from the traditional 7-day rotation to the rapidly rotating 'continental' (two-day) rota showed a rise in certified sickness of 36%, a rise in uncertified sickness absence of 29%, but a fall in the absence for other reasons of 2%.*

Research seems to be inconclusive, and perhaps the dominant factor is the social acceptability of the particular shift system.

Shift and Day Work

Shift workers seem no more prone to illness than those who have never worked on shifts. There is probably a certain amount of self-selection, as there appears to be a small proportion of people who cannot tolerate shift work and develop nervous or digestive disorders after a few days or weeks. Shift work becomes so unpleasant that they have to give it up.

Taylor studied sickness absence of male refinery workers over a 4-year period. His results showed that continuous three-cycle shift workers have consistently and significantly lower rates of sickness than day workers in similar occupations. He suggested that the main reasons for the difference lie in the degree of personal involvement in the work and in the social structure of the working group.†

Bibliography

Harrington J. M. (1978) *Shift Work and Health: A Critical Review of the Literature*. Health and Safety Executive. HMSO.
International Occupational Safety and Health Information Centre (CIS) (1965) Sheet No. 11. *Artificial Lighting in Factory and Office.*
Kellerman F. T., van Wely P. A. and Willems (1963) *Vademecum Ergonomics in Industry*. Philips Technical Library.

* Pocock S. J., Sergean R. and Taylor P. J. (1972) *Occupational Psychology*, **46**, 7–13.
† Taylor P. J. (1967) *Br. J. Ind. Med.* **24**, 93.

8

The Need for Observation

The environment in employment is not selected by the worker, but is determined by the particular trade or process. The observations of Ramazzini and Thackrah are classic in their relating occupational cause and effect. As industry becomes more complex and an increasing number of synthetic chemicals come into use, one cannot wait for the development of easily identifiable disease. The employer must be alert, observation must be refined, and relevant data should be collected.

Data Collection

Without prescience, how much data should be sought? Many studies have needed data on age, length of service (exposure), morbidity and mortality. These data are usually included in records of employment, sickness returns, pensions and death certificates. Good sickness and surgery attendance records can give an early clue to possible danger; the occurrence of a similar complaint in a group of workers will alert the physician to enquire further. It was in this way that acro-osteolysis due to vinyl chloride was discovered.

Epidemiology

Whilst a single observation may offer a clue, full proof of occupational cause may be difficult to establish. Some agents have a long latent period between exposure and effect. Others may produce a disease which occurs naturally, e.g. lung cancer, and definite increase in incidence has to be established. The disease experience of groups of workers has to be studied.

Epidemiology is a branch of medical science concerned with the study of the frequency and distribution of disease in defined populations. No disease is distributed regularly throughout a population, and the study of the irregularities has two aims: first, by relating the uneven distribution to environmental, personal, and temporal factors, to identify aetiological factors that may be controllable; second to provide information essential to the planning and delivery of health care services for the population.

In occupational medicine the main uses of epidemiology are:

1. To quantify known hazards, e.g. lung cancer in gas retort workers.

2. To search for causes, e.g. relationship between mesothelioma and asbestos exposure.

The techniques are:

1. Cohort study. A group of workers is matched by a group which is similar in every respect, except exposure, to whatever agent or process is to be considered. The morbidity or mortality experience of the two groups is then observed, either prospectively or retrospectively from previous records.

2. *Case control study.* In this study the starting point is the group which is affected, and there is an attempt to uncover possible causes. This is the classical epidemiological method, e.g. the observation of the occurrence of typhoid in those who drank a particular supply of water. The groups are studied retrospectively, one with the disease, the other without, and occupational causes are sought. Not all those who are exposed are affected to the same degree and if the exposure is the cause of the disease a dose response type of relationship will be evident. The careful selection of controls is essential, and the data observed must be subjected to statistical analysis to avoid drawing conclusions on findings that may occur by chance.

3. *Intervention study.* This type of study is concerned with measuring the effect on the health of a working population of controlling an occupational exposure suspected by means of cohort or case-control studies of being harmful to health. Final proof of a causal relationship between an occupational exposure and a particular disease is provided if the intervention eliminates or lowers substantially the incidence of the disease in the experimental population.

STATISTICS

Definition

The assembly, classification, tabulation and analysis of numerical data.

Objects

A statistical investigation should be concerned with a definite objective such as testing a hypothesis and before its commencement it is prudent to seek the advice of a medical statistician.

Measurement of Central Tendency. Medical information is quantified and for the present purpose each element is termed 'quantity'. Quantities which vary from the average are called variates and they are of two kinds. *Continuous variates* can have any value within a particular range (e.g. age, body weight, height). *Discontinuous* or *discrete variates* can have only isolated values, whole numbers (e.g. number of persons in a family).

The simplest way of expressing the representative quantity of a set of data of the same genus is by using a *measure of central tendency*. There are several of these and it is important that the appropriate one is used in a particular investigation.

1. The *arithmetic mean* is used where quantities are recorded in a set of observations; it is the sum of the quantities divided by the number of quantities. The *weighted mean* is used to average the averages of two or more sets of data; it is determined by summating the products of the average of each set by the number of observations in the set and dividing by the total number of observations in all the sets.

2. The *median* is the value of the middle quantity when all the quantities are arranged in order of magnitude.

3. The *mode* is the quantity which occurs most frequently in a series. It is the maximum point on the frequency distribution curve.

Frequency Distribution is the presentation of the data in a condensed form in terms of class intervals and frequencies (*Fig. 8.1*). It may take the form of a tabular statement or a diagram with the variate measured along the x axis (horizontal) and the frequency along the y axis (vertical).

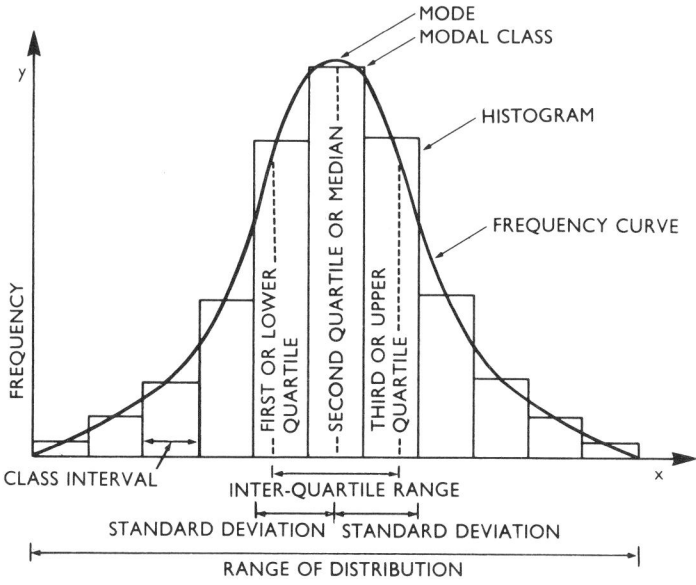

Fig. 8.1. Frequency distribution — normal curve.

Care is necessary in selecting the scales of the diagram so that the eye is not deceived. The area enclosed by the diagram represents the total frequency.

Diagrams take the form of:

Histogram or *bar chart* which consists of a series of rectangles or bars, with the width of each rectangle representing a class interval and the height the frequency of that class.

Frequency polygon where the frequency of each interval is plotted above the midpoint of the interval, and these points are joined together by straight lines.

Frequency curve where a smooth curve is drawn to fit as closely as possible the histogram or frequency polygon. It is the preferred method of representation as it is amenable to mathematical treatment. The extreme ends of the frequency curve are called *tails* and are ignored in some investigations.

The range, mode and median give a broad description of the data. Such numerical characteristics of the data are called *parameters*. In the 'normal' frequency distribution the mean, mode and median all coincide.

A finer description of the data is given by *quartiles*, which are those values of the variate which divide the frequency curve into four equal parts. The *first* or *lower quartile* applies to the lower part of the range, and the *third* or *upper quartile* to the upper part. Even finer definition is given by *deciles* (10 equal parts) and percentiles (100 equal parts).

The presentation shows at a glance:

The difference between the least and the greatest values of the variate, termed *range of distribution*.

The interval with the greatest frequency, the *mode* for discrete variates and *modal class* for continuous variates. Sometimes called the *norm*.

The spread of the frequencies, termed *dispersion of the distribution*, or *variance*.

In some investigations (e.g. heights of men) the distribution is fairly symmetrical with the mode at or near the centre of the range. This is called a normal curve and in such distributions the mean, the mode and the median coincide (*see below*). In other investigations (e.g. body weight) the mode is remote from the centre and the curve is said to be asymmetric or *skew*. *Positive skewness* is where the tail extends into the larger values of the variate; *negative skewness* is where it extends into the lesser values.

A frequency curve is usually *unimodal* but may be *multimodal* (two or more humps).

Other ways of presenting a set of data are *horizontal bar chart* and the *scatter diagram* where each individual value is plotted.

Frequency curve. It is unlikely that a series of observations of natural quantities will show perfect symmetry of frequency distribution. A number of theoretic distributions are available and the most useful one is the '*normal*', '*standard*' or *Gaussian curve*; this is used for dealing with quantities whose magnitude is continuously variable.

Deviation is the difference in value between a variate and the mean. Some deviations are positive, others negative. The *standard deviation* is a measure of scatter of a series of observations about the mean. A large SD indicates a wide scatter. If the differences were added, the positive would be balanced by the negative, so the squares of the differences are added, the sum is divided by the number of observations to give the mean of the squares, which is known as the *variance*. The square root of this gives the standard deviation, or root mean square deviation. For mathematical reasons a slightly better result is obtained by using the number of observations -1. The formula is:

$$\text{Standard deviation} = \sqrt{\frac{\Sigma\,(x - \bar{x})^2}{N - 1}}$$

where Σ = sum of
     x = each variate under observation
     $\bar{x}$ = the mean of all observations
     N = number of all observations.

The standard deviation is a convenient measure of the amount of scatter. It can be calculated that in normal frequency distribution, 68·27% of the observations lie within the standard deviation; 95·45% lie within 2× the standard deviation and 99·73% within 3× the standard deviation. In other words only 1 in about 20 observations will differ from the mean by more than 2× the standard deviation, and about 1 in 370 will differ from the mean by more than $3\times$ the standard deviation (plus or minus).

Significance is descriptive of a result which is very unlikely to arise by chance. *Tests of significance* are used to show whether the characteristics of the data are likely to have been caused by chance due to random variations within the data, or whether they are a peculiar characteristic.

The Chi-squared Test is used in testing association between grouped observations, e.g. smoking and lung cancer. It is essential to decide what part chance could have played in any result obtained. This test is carried out by finding how many observations vary from the expected findings if there were no relation between the characteristics under consideration. The differences between expected and observed findings are squared to remove any minus quantities and divided by expected finding. The chi-squared is given by the summation of all the values. It would be nought if the expected and observed results were similar. Inevitably it has some positive value, which is low if the differences could have arisen by chance and high if chance is unlikely to have influenced the findings significantly.

The chi-squared test is interpreted by the use of Fisher's tables which give the *probability*, symbolized by the letter P. Probability is expressed on a scale between 0 and 1, so that an impossible event has a probability of 0 and an event that is certain to occur has a probability of 1. If the value of P is 0·05 the differences observed would occur up to once in every twenty times by chance. P of 0·05 and less is usually regarded as 'significant'.

The T-test of significance is used where there is only a small number of observations, usually less than 30, when it cannot be assumed that the standard deviation is fully representative. The 't' value is the ratio of the observed difference between the means of two samples to the calculated standard error of that difference. The number of observations and the value of 't' allows the probability P to be read off from a special table.

Other Definitions

Correlation is the reciprocal or association between two sets of variables. The *coefficient of correlation* measures the closeness of the relationship. It has limiting values of $+1$ and -1. Positive values indicate direct dependence of one characteristic on the other and at $+1$ the dependence is complete. Negative values indicate inverse dependence, -1 that the inverse dependence is complete. *Multiple correlation* refers to the correlation of one variable with two others. *Partial correlation* refers to the correlation of two variables independently of a third variable.

Regression is the tendency to approach the average. *Regression analysis* is the study of two or more associated variables. *Regression equation* is a mathematical statement of how one variable depends upon another. *Regression line* of dependent variable on independent variable is a line of best fit when the independent variables are known accurately.

Sampling is a device for researching a large set of data by selecting a small part for study where it is uneconomic or impossible to investigate the whole set.

Sample is a small representative part of a whole; it is expressed as a fraction of the whole, e.g. 1 in 8.

Random sample is a sample chosen in such a way that all quantities in the set have a known chance of being included. Tables of random sampling numbers are available.

Stratified sample. Where the data to be sampled can be subdivided into subgroups each having distinct differences in the characteristic(s) under investigation, a random sample is taken from each subgroup to ensure that all subgroups are fairly represented in the sample.

Sampling error is the difference between the average of the sample and the average of a full investigation. Its amount depends on the size of the sample, the variability of the data and the way in which the sample is chosen.

Standard error is calculated by dividing the standard deviation of the quantities in a sample by the square root of the number of quantities in the sample. It is a measure of how far a sample value is likely to differ from the true value. Not applicable to very small samples and should be used with caution in samples of less than 100 quantities.

Expectation is the degree of probability of a certain event taking place.

MORTALITY AND MORBIDITY DATA

Mortality

Mortality data are useful in relating occupation to risk in disease of fatal consequence, e.g. cancer. Care in interpretation is needed, as the occupation stated at the registration of a death is the last one of the individual, and this may give no indication of the main occupation during his working life. Detailed enquiries may be needed to establish a full occupational history. In England and Wales the Registrar-General published decennial supplements to his statistical reviews, which include statistics of occupational mortality. Occupational mortality can be compared by using the Standardized Mortality Ratio (SMR) (*Table 8.1*). The SMR is the number of actual deaths given as a percentage of the expected deaths. Expected deaths in each group are calculated by applying the age specific national death rates to the population studied.

Morbidity

The inaccuracies, sometimes deliberate, in completing sickness certificates make this form of morbidity data very unreliable. Sickness records kept at the workplace may be more accurate, and they often lead to the identification of a hazard. For example, the occurrence of dermatitis in a group of workers will lead to an investigation of the tasks involved and the methods of work.

Sickness Absence. Absenteeism in industry disrupts the smooth running of the enterprise and places a burden on other workers. It is natural that a firm appointing a doctor should expect some improvement in its sickness absence

Table 8.1. Some occupational variations (Office of Population Censuses and Surveys (1978), *Occupational Mortality, Decennial Supplement* 1970–72. London, HMSO DS No. 1)

Occupation	SMR — all causes	SMR — some specific causes
Fishermen	171	Accidents 253
Foundry labourers	163	Respiratory disease 278
Coal miners	141	Respiratory disease 252, Accidents 156
Policemen	109	Circulatory disease 131
Agricultural workers	101	Accidents 155
Firemen	99	Accidents 81 Respiratory 61
Postmen	81	
Teachers	66	
Local government senior officers	57	

These figures should be interpreted with caution e.g. firemen and policemen usually retire by the age of 55 and then take up a new occupation. The statistics, and the excellent critical analysis should be studied in full.

experience. Nevertheless, it would be unwise for the occupational physician to foster this belief. It is an unfortunate fact that the inauguration of an occupational health service has been shown repeatedly to have little or no impact on sickness absence figures.

The explanation is that sickness absence statistics are not an accurate mirror of the state of health of the work force. The causes of absence are complex, and only relatively minor ones (such as 'preventive' treatment at the place of work) lie within the control of the works medical department. It is preferable to speak of 'absence attributed to sickness' rather than 'sickness absence'.

Definition 1. Sickness absence is absence from work accepted by the employer as attributable to sickness or accident (*Table 8.2*).

Table 8.2. Days lost through sickness per insured employed person in England and Wales

Year	Days lost
1955	12
1965	14·5
1974	16·6
1983	15

Advances in medicine have rendered many diseases treatable; with the advent of the welfare state medical and social care has greatly improved. Despite this there had been a steady rise in sickness absence, mostly short-term until 1983. There are many factors which may account for this paradox, including the higher expectations of the individual and improved insurance benefits.

In 1964 300 million working days were lost through sickness in England and Wales, some of the major causes are given in *Table 8.3.*

Some factors influencing sickness absence

1. Absence Prone. 70% of insured workers have no spells of absence in any one year, 25% have one spell, 2% have three spells or more.

2. Age.

16 years to 20 years: 6 days/man/year.

60 years to 64 years: 42 days/man/year.

Table 8.3.   Some major causes of sickness absence

	Million days/year
Bronchitis	30
Cardiovascular disease	30
Rheumatic diseases	25
Psychosomatic diseases	25
Industrial accidents	20
Prescribed industrial diseases	1·5

3. Size of Working Group. Comparative studies have shown that in smaller concerns where the individual has a greater sense of his own worth, fewer man-days per head are lost than in larger enterprises; this is also true of some small units in larger enterprises, where there is a strong sense of cohesion in the working group.

4. Morale. Frequent short spells of absences are often seen in working groups where there is poor morale. Short-term absences are in fact an index of the individual's sense of the significance of his work and his identification with the objects of the enterprise — in other words, an index of morale.

5. Regional. There is a large geographical variation in average absence, and this is not always related to industrialization. The sickness absenteeism in Wales is 151%, West Midlands 95%, S.E. England 76% of the national average.

6. Social Factors. Social background and home circumstances are among the non-medical factors found to be related to sickness absence. If work is tedious and monotonous and the worker feels that he is looked on as being of little account, feeling indisposed will be taken as a legitimate reason for a day off, whereas the tendency will be for a managing director, a self-employed person or a professional man whose tasks are all felt to carry responsibility, to come to work if he possibly can. This is not to accuse the shop-floor worker of malingering (which is fairly rare but not unknown). It really reflects the failure of modern industrial production and of some present-day managements to ensure that the worker's capacity is used sufficiently fully, and that he feels his own importance in the scheme of things. The same factor will tend to prolong the period taken off for many minor illnesses. Experiments in 'job enrichment' which are being tried in the car assembly plants of Volvo and Saab aim to do this by reorganizing production so as to give increased responsibility to small working groups.

It is interesting to note that shift workers have been found to have consistently less absence than day workers and that overtime working is not associated with high absenteeism. On the other hand, there is some evidence that absence is higher in those whose journey to work is inconvenient or difficult.*

Definition 2. Accepting that there are many factors influencing sickness absence, particularly where there is no serious morbidity, we could offer another definition: Sickness absence is absence for which sickness is made the excuse.

Attitudes to sickness absence
1. The patient; it may be:
   An excuse — a deliberate abstention from work.
   An escape — psychosomatic symptoms withdrawing him from an unpleasant environment.
   A nuisance — a true illness which necessitates his absence from work.

* Taylor P. J. (1974) *J. R. Coll. Physicians Lond.* **8**, 315.

2. The doctor. Absence from work may be a necessary part of treatment, a certificate is issued when the patient presents for advice. The end of the absence need not be so definite, and many factors, including the patient, may influence the length of absence.

In true disease, the doctor recognizes the need to issue a certificate, but he takes an unfavourable view of managements which demand that a worker absenting himself for trivial or non-existent health reasons should obtain a doctor's certificate.

3. The employer. In demanding certificates for absence due to sickness, the employer creates a situation where an employee can justify his absence by producing a certificate. When the employer feels that workers are absenting themselves unnecessarily (and they may even be taking it in turn to have a few days 'on the sick') he feels powerless to do anything because the absence is certified by a doctor. The employer may even welcome the assumption that the responsibility to tackle the problem is taken from him. Failing to take normal managerial action, all he does is to blame the certifying doctor.

Some measures of control

1. Firms which operate sickness payments from the first day of absence should remove from the general practitioner the burden of certifying for a short spell (1–3 day) absences. These form nearly 15% of sickness absenteeism. A system of self-certification by the worker introduced at an oil refinery* was not abused; short absences were spread evenly throughout the week, instead of clustering at week-ends. Similar measures introduced in another industry showed that the number of short absences increased, but the total absenteeism remained constant.

2. Management must accept responsibility for dealing with absenteeism. There is no reason why employees with bad records should not be interviewed. Those who are truly ill, and may need some help, will not resent this measure. Sometimes welfare and social problems are disclosed in this way. If a manager complains to an industrial doctor about high sickness absence rates, the doctor should first ask the manager what he has done about it.

3. In serious illness or injury, the industrial doctor should consult the general practitioner, and offer help during the stage of recovery. This is discussed in the section on rehabilitation. (Chapter 6.)

4. There is some value in certification, especially in the more important diseases, as a basis for morbidity studies. The ILO Recommendation 112 states: 'Occupational Health Services should not be precluded from obtaining information about a worker's illness, so that they will be better able to evaluate their preventive programme, discover occupational hazards, and recommend the suitable placement of workers for rehabilitation purposes'.

The study of absence attributed to sickness is one of the functions of the occupational physician, and in a large concern the varying experience of different sections and departments may give important pointers both to the possibility of environmental factors playing a part, and to the morale. It is customary for the doctor to see employees returning after long-term sickness — usually three weeks or more. This enables him to decide whether a change of job is called for, either permanently or until recovery is complete. Moreover, the early symptoms of many occupational illnesses are non-specific, and may not suggest an occupational cause to the general practitioner who sees only the isolated case; but a high

* Taylor P. J. (1969) *Br. Med. J.* **1**, 144–7.

incidence of, for example, symptoms of respiratory illness in one section of a factory may well call for investigation of the working environment.

Sickness absence data

1. *Measurement of frequency*

    Inception rate (Spells of absence)

    $$= \frac{\text{Number of episodes of absence in a year}}{\text{Average population at risk during year}}$$

    Inception rate (Persons)

    $$= \frac{\text{Number of persons having one or more episodes in a year}}{\text{Average population at risk}}$$

    Point prevalence rate

    $$= \frac{\text{Number of persons absent on a day}}{\text{Population at risk on the day}}$$

2. *Measures of severity*

    Annual duration per person

    $$= \frac{\text{Number of days lost in a year}}{\text{Average population at risk during year}}$$

    Lost-time percentage

    $$= \frac{\text{Number of working days (or hours) lost} \times 100}{\text{Total normal potential working days (or hours)}}$$

    Average length of spell

    $$= \frac{\text{Number of days lost}}{\text{Number of episodes}}$$

Sickness Calendar. In addition to the more detailed sickness records, a very useful device is for each local manager to keep a separate annual calendar for each employee. Each day of absence is ticked off on this calendar; short-term absence patterns, and total absenteeism, can readily be observed.

Self-certified Sickness. Since 1983 employees have been able to self-certify sickness for up to 7 days. This avoids their having to bother their general practitioners for sick notes for trivial illnesses, it avoids a great deal of administrative cost and it also enables the employer to monitor more readily short-term sickness absenteeism.

Since the same date employers have also been responsible for paying the first eight weeks of sickness benefit — so-called 'Statutory Sick Pay'. Employers are required to pay a flat rate of benefit to employees, no National Insurance Benefits are payable. The scheme provides for compensation for employers for this liability. This measure also enhances the employers' awareness of sickness absenteeism and should lead to better monitoring.

Bibliography

Manpower Papers. No. 4. Absenteeism. Department of Employment. London, HMSO.
Principles of Medical Statistics. Sir Austin Bradford Hill. London, The Lancet Ltd.
Proceedings of Symposium on Absence from Work Attributed to Sickness. Society of Occupational Medicine.

Chapter 9 — Industrial Psychology and Mental Health

Human Relations at Work

The master and servant relationship is no longer appropriate as industrial organizations have grown in size and complexity. The owner is no longer the boss, or direct leader. People with professional and technical skills find themselves in positions of management, and workers become organized into groups. The systematic study of human relationships in industry is relatively new, sometimes viewed with suspicion by managers who think they know all about it, and by workers who suspect they may be manipulated by a clever and sinister new tool of management. Yet industry increasingly relies upon skill rather than brute force. In addition to technical skills, people need to be taught skills in management, we need satisfaction from work, good leadership and team-work, a sense of achievement and belonging. From practical experience, managers, industrial doctors and nurses have some knowledge of human relationships in industry, but they can benefit from a systematic study of the subject. Industrial psychology has developed greatly in the last few decades, and the industrial psychologist can bring many useful skills into the study of human relations.

Staff Selection

Industrial psychology was originally limited to the application of special psychological tests to help with staff selection. Measurements of intelligence, vocational achievement, aptitude and sometimes personality, can be very useful in selecting applicants for certain tasks. People with a high score on obsessional factors of personality are better placed in routine repetitive tasks, or those which require vigilance. Some people on the borderline of subnormal intelligence can present as intellectually bright until formally tested; this could be disastrous if the job required intelligence. These tests can be particularly helpful when dealing with difficult cases for re-deployment. Most people find their own careers satisfactorily, either by themselves or with the help of Careers and Youth Employment Officers, but an enforced change of career due to illness or industrial change can be very difficult. Counselling will be far more effective when it is supported by knowledge of the individual's abilities and aptitudes. In one industry which went through a very great change and many redundancies, it was found that many workers were capable of tackling more difficult and better paid jobs.

Job Analysis

To advise on correct placement, the industrial psychologist has to have a description of the job. Some early work in industrial psychology involved the detailed *analysis* of jobs. By closely studying the operations required in certain description of the job. Some early work in industrial psychology involved the detailed *analysis* of jobs. By closely studying the operations required in certain jobs, it became evident that the traditional methods were wasteful of energy and poorly productive.

Staff Training

Many firms have set up their own training departments, providing courses in communication, interviewing, counselling, etc. There are also some business training schools, sandwich courses at universities, and management training colleges to which middle and senior management can be sent. These have the advantage of highly professional instruction in up-to-date skills, but there may sometimes be a disadvantage in that the student has difficulty in reconciling his new academic knowledge to the rough and tumble of the practical situation at work.

Man and Work

'What is work? Work is of two kinds: first, altering the position of matter at or near the earth's surface relatively to other such matter; second, telling other people to do so. The first kind is unpleasant and ill-paid; the second is pleasant and highly paid. The second kind is capable of indefinite extension: there are not only those who give orders, but those who give advice as to what orders should be given. Usually two opposite kinds of advice are given simultaneously by two organized bodies of men; this is called politics.' (Bertrand Russell: *In Praise of Idleness*.)

Since Bertrand Russell wrote that in 1932, much has changed, although the cynicism remains. There is less work in the purely physical sense, and as automation progresses there will be even less. As there is less direct sense of achievement in actually making something with one's own hands, what are the factors which are important in work?

Hawthorne Experiment

In 1938 Whitehead described an experiment in the Hawthorne Works of the Western Electric Company in the USA. The experiment showed that output increased when the conditions of work were improved following discussion with the workers. However, the increased output continued when they returned to the original imperfect conditions. The discussions and involvement with the workforce had a greater effect on their morale than their physical conditions at work.

Motivation – Hygiene Theory

Herzberg maintains that employees are not motivated by improving work conditions, raising salaries or shuffling tasks 'if I kick my dog he will move. When I want him to move again, what must I do? I must kick him again. Similarly, I can charge a man's battery and then re-charge it and re-charge it again. But it is only when he has his own generator that we can talk about motivation. He then needs no outside stimulation. He wants to do it'. Ever increasing pay demands in certain industries illustrate the point that pay never satisfies, and it does not contribute to self-motivation. Herzberg, in his motivation – hygiene theory, describes two groups of factors. He points out that the opposite of dissatisfaction is not necessarily satisfaction. Motivators are factors which give job satisfaction, hygiene factors are those which remove certain areas of dissatisfaction. These two groups of factors are entirely different. The five strong motivating factors for job satisfaction are achievement, recognition, the work itself, responsibility and advancement; the last three being of greatest importance for lasting change of attitudes. The major dissatisfiers are company policy and administration, supervision, salary, inter-personal relations and working conditions.

Job Enrichment

It follows that by concentrating on the motivators, particularly the three outstanding ones, there should be a profound effect on motivation. This is called job enrichment. A simple illustration is the removal of a single repetitive task from a production line, and organizing a group of workers into a team who will carry out the complete assembly of a vehicle. This has been tried by one of the major motor manufacturers, but evidence has not convinced everyone of the success of this measure. However, there are simple measures which can be used and which are usually effective: involving the workers in decision making, suggestion schemes, and by discussing company results.

Change

There is often a resistance to change. This applies especially to old established industries which have evolved over many years. Each person has a place and a function to fulfil, and rigid lines of demarcation are developed. This further prevents adaptation to change, sometimes even when industrial survival is in question. The fear of change is not new, for in the middle of the industrial revolution the Luddites smashed the new machines for the hosiery trade.

Counselling

This is one of the management techniques now taught in staff training programmes, but it is worthy of special mention. One specific use of counselling in management is for *management appraisal*. This provides a formal structure whereby there is a regular appraisal interview, usually annually, between the manager and his superior. It allows for a discussion of aims and achievement, and it may be used to identify potential candidates for promotion. Necessarily, this technique only applies to the middle and to higher levels of management.

A more general form of counselling can be used at all levels of management, and although it may be less formal, at least it does mean that each manager sets aside sufficient time to talk with each of his immediate subordinates.

Crisis

There may specific occasions where special counselling may be needed. This will apply especially if there are to be any major changes in the work, or if there are to be redundancies. Here the theory of *crisis intervention* is useful. Crisis refers to the person's emotional reaction to a hazardous situation, not to the situation itself. In a crisis the individual goes through a phase of disturbance and turmoil during which he shows dependency, suggestibility, and a need to talk about his problems. After a matter of a few weeks he will achieve some form of adaptation, although this may be of a maladaptive or neurotic nature. During the crisis situation the individual has a state of heightened suggestibility, for better or worse. Well directed and helpful counselling at this stage, taking into account the subject's personality, will help him to find a satisfactory solution. Without this intervention he may well fall prey to misguided advice from barrack room lawyer agitation.

The counsellor should be aware of the disturbances that can occur in crisis, people's reactions may be quite at variance with their usual personality. Gross reactions may vary from intense over-caution with concentration on trivia to blustering self-confidence or even aggression.

Stress in Industry

Recently, there has been considerable thought given to stress in management. There is no satisfactory definition of stress; Hans Selye defines it as a non-specific response of the body to any demand made on it. Occupational stress could be caused by physical and mental demands, but physical factors such as heat or physical workload are related to well understood physical stresses. This discussion of stress in industry is confined to the psychological stresses which occur, particularly at management levels. In industry, stress may be made evident directly as illness, or indirectly as absenteeism, accidents, conflicts and misjudgements. Additionally, people with emotional difficulties use only a part of their possible capabilities. Stress may particularly occur at times of change when there is need to adapt to new conditions. Large numbers of work people can be involved with major industrial changes and closures.

In one large industry facing partial closure, a general health questionnaire was administered to the workforce. This showed a twofold increase in abnormal scores (i.e. above the threshold of mental illness) of those who were facing redundancy. It also helped to identify individuals who would need particular care with counselling. Even in those whose jobs were secure, there were 5 per cent who appeared to have a constitutional tendency to suffer from more severe continuous symptoms.

Insecurity giving rise to stress can stem from over-stretching with too many demands either in quality or quantity, under-stretching and frustration, boring work, deprivation of work satisfaction, or changes at work. A number of breakdowns in middle age are due to the imposition of organizational change at a time when the individual's power of adaptation is declining.

Stress in Management

At a time when there are increasing demands on managers, financial controls, marketing, computers, behavioural sciences, research and development programmes, etc. there is also a fall in managers' prestige. Managers are made to feel inferior to politicians who can demand performance but remove the facilities. At present management have five major worries: inflation, government interference, disobedient workers, difficult union negotiations, and adverse social climate. Managers are learning to cope with the better educated and more eloquent workforce, to be less authoritative and more liberal: this adaptation should help to reduce stress.

The organization can certainly contribute to managerial stress, particularly when there is imposition of overload, manpower reductions reduce the ability to delegate, and communications and human relations are poor.

Stress and Heart Disease

In the UK there is little evidence that executives have a special risk of heart disease. In the Civil Service the incidence of ischaemic heart disease in the lower clerical grades is twice that in the higher grades.

The high catecholamine release in stress is biologically appropriate for immediate activity; but this 'stone age' biochemical mechanism becomes dangerous when there is no exertion to metabolize the fats released to the bloodstream or to reduce the blood pressure. These dangerous effects are augmented by cigarette smoking and over-eating. Doctors and other professional people have markedly reduced their cigarette smoking during the last 20 years. Unfortunately there has not been such a significant trend in the social classes IV and V.

Mental Illness

It has been estimated that in any one year between 10 and 20% of a general practitioner's patients will suffer a minor psychiatric illness. Major psychiatric illnesses are much less frequent, severe depression occurring in about 0·5% of adult patients each year. With so much minor psychiatric illness occurring it is inevitable that there will be some problems in employment. The major psychiatric illnesses will require some urgent treatment, but they are not necessarily a bar to employment. Apart from those with severe organic psychoses, most psychiatric patients are employable, though sometimes special arrangements are needed.

Despite the very common occurrence of psychiatric illness, there is still a great deal of prejudice about it. In a recent case that came to an industrial trial tribunal an employee had been dismissed because he had eventually disclosed a history of a minor mental illness. He had worked successfully, with commendation, but his employer maintained that had he disclosed his previous history at the time of recruitment, he would not have been accepted for employment.

In his book *Something Happened* Joseph Heller illustrates the fear and prejudice about mental illness...

'and there is one typist in our department who is going crazy slowly and has all of us afraid of her.... Our biggest fear is that she will go crazy on a weekday between 9·00 and 5·00. We hope she will go crazy on a weekend, when we aren't with her. We should get her out of the company now, while there is still time. But we won't. Somebody should fire her; nobody will. Even Green, who actually enjoys firing people, recoils from the responsibility of making the move that might bring about her shattering collapse, although he cannot stand her, detests the way she looks and is infuriated by every reminder that she still exists in his department.'

Management of Mental Ill Health

Mental illness is often not detected because of its insidious onset. In depression the patient will often show social withdrawal, becoming morose and sullen with his workmates and showing a marked lack of self-confidence. In a paranoid disorder he may show increased sensitivity, secretiveness and suspicious behaviour. There is a better chance of these patients being brought to the doctor early when the medical service enjoys a good rapport and confidence with the workforce.

With minor psychiatric illness the symptoms may be just as tiresome to his workmates as they are to the patient, particularly if he works in a small group. But the individual's colleagues or his superior can often help by rendering mental first aid.

Someone who has the skill to listen without emotionally reacting to the patient and who can give sound, practical commonsense advice, can be of great help. The industrial doctor, nurse, or skilful personnel officer can deal with a breakdown and get the patient to skilled help at a very early stage. Where the problem becomes persistent or repeated, the working group will lose patience, morale will drop, and eventually the patient will become isolated and rejected. If the illness affects the work then the patient's career will be threatened. Whilst the sufferer needs practical help, understanding and sympathy, he also has the right of access to normal management procedures, including disciplinary measures and appeals. It is wrong to shield the employee with a mental illness, for it may well delay his seeking professional advice and treatment, and it will not help management to apply correct remedial action. Most organizations have a 'disciplinary procedure'. This is misnamed; it is more a management code of practice, for it helps as well as disciplines. The procedure, with interviews, warnings and appeals is as much for the protection of the employee as it is for the convenience of management.

In mental illness, excepting in the organic psychoses, no organic aetiology has been found, neither is there any demonstrable pathology. The diagnosis mainly rests upon the difference in behaviour between the individual and the rest of the community — it is an 'operational definition'. If an individual's behaviour is so different from that which is expected it should be made clear to him. This point is well illustrated by the case of a social worker who displayed some psychiatric symptoms. Instead of improving the relationships with the community he positively hindered them. His behaviour was unpredictable and at times aggressive. He was offered alternative employment away from contact with the public. He refused this offer and was dismissed. He appealed against his dismissal and at the industrial tribunal the exact psychiatric label that could be attached to his behaviour was not relevant. What was held to be relevant was the unacceptable behaviour, and the management were asked for clear accounts of this.

Alcoholism

It has been estimated that alcoholism occurs in between 3 and 20% of adult workers. There are some occupational associations with alcoholism. There are relatively high rates of alcoholism in company directors, brewery workers, seamen and waiters; almost directly proportional to the ease of access to alcohol. If the sufferer is to be helped it must be done at an early stage, when it is extremely difficult to identify him, and he would not regard himself as a 'sufferer'. Early signs are: extended lunch hour, lack of concentration in the afternoons, eventually extending all day, lateness or absenteeism on Mondays, deterioration in work, deterioration in personal appearance and habits. Very often these people are sheltered by their workmates and the condition is not identified until it has reached serious proportions, when security of employment is threatened.

Alcoholism Policy. It is advisable for employers to reach agreement with employees and Trade Unions, on a company alcoholism policy. If alcoholism is to be recognized and treated at an early stage the alcoholic must be identified early. He must not be sheltered by his workmates or management. A great deal of health education must be done to explain to all employees that they will do harm by not bringing the alcoholic to treatment early. An alcoholism policy should therefore commence with the education of the work force and management. The rest of the policy should include the following points:

1. Any employee who is thought to be suffering from alcoholism must be given the opportunity immediately to seek diagnosis and treatment. Whilst line managers or union representatives may recognize symptoms and signs which might be caused by alcoholism they are not in a position to confirm the diagnosis or to arrange treatment. These functions should be undertaken by the occupational health team who will arrange for the employee to receive the best possible advice and treatment. All these arrangements will only be made with the employee's express consent.

2. Whilst the employee is undergoing treatment he is considered to be on sick leave, if necessary, and is entitled to whatever sickness benefits are normally provided.

3. Every effort will be made to ensure that the employee, after treatment, is able to return to the same job which was held prior to treatment, unless his capacity has been affected to such an extent that resumption of the same job would be impossible or would lead to a serious risk of undermining satisfactory recovery.

4. If the employee cannot return to the same job, every effort should be made to redeploy him within the company. The general principle should be maintained that no demotion or retribution will occur unless matters of discipline are involved.

5. For employees who are nearing the end of their term of employment, or where it is considered more appropriate, the option of early retirement should be offered with full normal pension rights.

6. Employees who are thought to be suffering from alcoholism and who decline to accept referral for diagnosis and treatment, or who discontinue a course of treatment before its satisfactory completion and who continue with an unsatisfactory level of job performance will be subject to the normal and recognized disciplinary procedures.

7. The confidential nature of any records of employees with alcoholism or other health or social problems will be strictly preserved.

8. The policy is applicable to all employees, irrespective of the position which they hold, and there will be no discrimination at any level.

Epilepsy

Although epilepsy presents certain physical restrictions on employment, it is mentioned here because more often it is the behavioural problems which provide the greater difficulty in employment. There is still much prejudice concerning employment of epileptics, and very often the patient's own doctor will advise him not to declare the fact that he is epileptic. This is very short-sighted, because when it becomes obvious his employer than accuses him of dishonesty and his job is threatened. For those whose attacks are well controlled there are very few restrictions on employment, but there is an absolute bar for bus or heavy goods vehicle driving. It is wise to warn the working group that an attack may occur, and to give some simple advice on how the patient should be helped. It is often much more difficult for the working group to understand the emotional irregularities of the epileptic, who may display moods of resentment, excitability, or even aggression.

Employment of the Mentally Ill

Those employees who suffer an acute mental illness can usually be rehabilitated back to their normal jobs after appropriate treatment. With chronic mental illness very careful placement is necessary, but it is often successfully made in a small working group where there is good supervision by a sensitive and understanding management. Where more specific supervision is needed, the mentally sick can be employed in special groups either within a factory (often in the care of a mental nurse) or within a sheltered workshop which will do work for various factories on a contract basis. Those who are not well enough to be employed in normal competitive industry, or in an industrial therapy workshop, usually have some employment in special centres in the industrial therapy departments of the larger mental hospitals. This category is almost entirely confined to those who have been in mental hospital for a long time and have become institutionalized.

Modern drugs have greatly changed the prognosis in mental illness, and many more patients are able to return to normal work in industry. Some former long-stay patients have been successful in obtaining and holding down jobs in industry. It is now accepted that groups working under supervision in open industry are superior to sheltered workshops in the management and re-training of the disabled. Early* reports a scheme in Bristol which has been run successfully for 12 years.

Sometimes the prognosis given by the psychiatrist proves to be over-optimistic. Whilst many patients with chronic mental illness can be employed, great care is needed with their placement and supervision. Repeated sickness absences or odd behaviour in one member of a small working group will be difficult to tolerate and may lead the group to show hostility, however well intentioned they may be at first. Usually these patients react very badly to stress, and they require relatively quiet, unharassing, unchanging jobs within a stable working group.

Retirement

Most of adult life is spent at work, and after 45 years of work there is a sudden and profound change on the day of retirement. Many industries now feel there is a moral obligation to help their workers to prepare for this change, and during their last year of work the employees are encouraged to attend pre-retirement courses. Industries which cannot provide these courses can use the ones provided by local Adult Education Centres. Along with the information on pensions and finance, a

* Early D. F. (1975) *Lancet* 1, 1370.

very important aspect is the change in life-style, the enjoyment of various leisure activities, health in later life, and the psychological adjustments required.

Bibliography

Health for Old Age and Arrangement for Old Age. (1972) Consumers Association.
Herzberg J. (1968) *Work and the Nature of Man.* St Albans, Crosby Lockwood.
Tredgold R. J. (1963) *Human Relations in Modern Industry.* London, Duckworth.

Chapter 10 — Women at Work

by Susan Robson

At present women make up almost 40% of the work force within the United Kingdom, but this has not always been the case.

Before the 15th Century women's work was concentrated on the home. With the growing development of the home weaving industry women and also children became involved in sorting, washing and spinning the wool whilst men were concerned solely with the weaving.

The results of this home-based industry were a source of cheap British goods for export and the rapid emergence of the wealthy middle classes, their fortunes dependent on trade.

In the 17th Century small mills and factories were developing dependent on trade, but the major industrial change came in the late 18th century, with the Industrial Revolution. Women and young children were employed in large numbers in the new factories and also in intolerable conditions in the coal mines.

The Census of 1841 showed six women's occupations: dressmaking, millinery, domestic science, agricultural labour, laundry and factory work. It was the conditions of women and children factory and mine workers which shocked the Victorians.

The Factories Act of 1844 promoted by Lord Shaftesbury banned the employment of women and girls underground and also included limitation on the hours of work to cover women for the first time.

In the Early 20th Century the scope of women's employment gradually widened with shop and office work giving better paid alternatives to domestic and factory labour.

World War I. At this time of National Emergency women were employed in almost every occupation normally followed by men. Protective legislation was put aside with the employment of women in what were previously purely men's occupations. During the 1914–1918 War more than one million women were involved in all areas of work, excluding underground mines.

1918. Women of 30 years and above were given the vote, but were expected to return from their wartime employment to their more traditional domestic roles.

World War II, 1939–1945. There was again an increased demand for women's labour, especially in the factories.

1961–1975. In the post-war era of full employment and industrial expansion there was increasing debate concerning the abolition of restrictions on women's work, culminating in a number of Acts of Parliament.

LEGISLATION AFFECTING WOMEN AT WORK

Present-day legislation concerning women at work is covered by the following.

1. The Equal Pay Act 1970. This Act came into force in 1975. Its purpose is to eliminate discrimination between men and women in regard to pay and other terms of employment.

2. The Sex Discrimination Act 1975. Applying to Great Britain but not Northern Ireland. It makes sex discrimination unlawful in employment, training and related matters, in education, in the provision of goods, facilities and services and in the disposal and management of premises. The Act gives individuals the right of direct access to the civil courts and industrial tribunals for legal remedies for unlawful discrimination.

3. The Employment Protection Act 1976. Among a number of provisions this gave an employee who is expecting a baby four rights:
   a. Not to be unreasonably refused time off for antenatal care and to be paid when permitted that time off.
   b. To complain of unfair dismissal because of pregnancy.
   c. To receive maternity pay (April 1977).
   d. To return to work with her employer after a period of absence on account of pregnancy or confinement.
   (There are some limitations as to eligibility.)

4. The Congenital Disabilities Act 1976. This provides that an employer may be sued by a child who is born disabled where it is believed that the disablement was caused by exposure to a reproductive toxin at the workplace. This implies that the employer has a duty to the unborn child both before and after conception. There is no duty on the employer if the child is not born alive.

5. Protective Legislation Concerned with the Hours of Work of Women
   a. The Hours of Employment Act 1936.
   b. The Mines and Quarries Act 1954.
   c. The Factories Act 1961.
   These acts contain legislation restructuring the working hours of women and children.
   Women's daily working hours are restricted to 9, weekly hours to 48.

Women's work spells to be not more than 4½ hours without a ½ hour break, or 5 hours if a 10 minute interval is given within this time.

Night work prohibited for women.

Most shift systems are also forbidden or restricted for women. There are, however, specific exemptions to the restrictions and there is provision for exemption from the requirements.

Sunday employment for women is prohibited.

The Equal Opportunities Commission has suggested that employers find the present system of restrictions unnecessary, bureaucratic and irksome, and a barrier to equal pay and job opportunities for women.

6. The Code of Practice: Lead at Work 1980. It is stated that: in order to safeguard the fetus:

a. A woman of reproductive capacity should be suspended if her blood lead exceeds 40 μg/100 ml.

b. She must immediately notify her supervisor if she suspects she is pregnant.

c. EMAS or an appointed doctor must be informed once pregnancy is suspected and on the advice of EMAS or the appointed doctor the woman may be suspended from work which exposes her to lead.

7. The Ionizing Radiation (Unsealed Radioactive Substances) Regulations 1968; The Ionizing Radiation (Sealed Radioactive Substances) Regulations 1969

a. The maximum permitted dose for a female in a quarter = 1·3 REM (13 mille sieverts).

b. If there is a suspicion of pregnancy the maximum dose to the abdomen during the remainder of pregnancy should not exceed 1 REM (10 mille sieverts).

8. The Public Health Act 1936. This prohibits the employment of a woman in a factory within 4 weeks of childbirth.

STATISTICS: WOMEN IN THE WORKING POPULATION

	1982 Males	1982 Females
United Kingdom Total Population	26·6m	28·1m
As a percentage of the total population of 54·7m	48·5%	51·5%

Trends over Time
Married women as % of labour force:

1921	1951	1961	1971	1981
3·8%	11·8%	16·3%	23·1%	25·9%

Earnings of Husbands and Wives
Where husband and wife both go out to work as employees:

1980 — 8%   of wives earned as much as or more than their husbands
1977 — 8%   of wives earned as much as or more than their husbands
1968 — 3½% of wives earned as much as or more than their husbands

Maternity Leave
Of 54% of women who worked during pregnancy and had the right of reinstatement, 10% took advantage of these rights and returned. In the public sector 25% of those who had the right to return took advantage of this right and returned to work.

Length of Working Life
It has been estimated that on average women are likely to be out of employment for a total of about seven years whilst establishing a family. This accounts for 16–19% of the time between 20 years and 59 years. Women's working lives are thus reduced but not dramatically curtailed.

COMPARISON OF THE PHYSICAL AND PSYCHOLOGICAL CHARACTERISTICS OF WOMEN AND MEN

With recent anti-discrimination legislation and the move towards equality, more women are moving into what have been traditionally considered male strongholds of employment.

Structural differences can be demonstrated between the average man and the average woman. However, the range of individual variability is very wide and this results in a degree of overlapping of physical characteristics and abilities between the sexes.

1. Strength. From an early age boys are stronger per unit body weight than girls of the same age.

2. Muscle. Anatomists and physiologists argue as to whether there are differences in the muscles between the sexes. Some biochemical differences have been demonstrated. Muscles are larger in males and enlargement is greater with training.

3. Growth. Growth of females is 2·2 years ahead of males. The growth period in males extends over a longer period (12–17 years) and usually results in greater height and weight. The average adult male is 20–25% heavier than the average adult female.

4. Respiratory (Aerobic Capacity)

a. Lung volumes in females are 10% smaller on average (even allowing for differences in body size).

b. Aerobic capacity (the maximum capability of an individual to utilize oxygen during physical exertion). If major factors are equal, i.e. training, age, height etc., then females may well have the same aerobic capacity as men.

5. Cardiovascular System. Average females have smaller hearts than average males. Maximum heart rate of females is 10% more than males: helping to offset the influence of the smaller heart on maximum cardiac output.

6. Visual. Men have better unaided visual acuity than women, especially distant vision. Defective colour vision is more common in men (1·88–12·8%).

7. Auditory. Hearing of men has been demonstrated at different frequencies to be inferior to that of women.

Age 20 years this is demonstrated at 4096 Hz and above.

Age 40 years this is demonstrated at 2048 Hz and above.

8. Strength

Male strength maximum — late 20s and remains so for 10 years; at 40 years is 95% maximum; at 50 years is 80% maximum.

Female strength maximum — early 20s and remains so for 10 years; at 30 years is 2/3 that of males same age; at 50 years is ½ that of males same age.

Strength declines more rapidly in women than men.

Males and females of the same age, build and physical fitness appear to have the same potential for physical work: an employer cannot therefore assume that any male will be capable of performing a task; neither must he or she presume that any female will be incapable.

GENERAL INFORMATION ON WORKING WOMEN

Books of only 20 years ago at a time of full employment now read like history. There have been some profound changes since the beginning of this century when social reformers were looking forward to the time when no married women need work.

Causes of Change

1. The pattern of family life: The move towards smaller families and easily available contraception.

2. Mechanization in the home.

3. Removal of social taboos: it is now considered respectable and even positively encouraged for women to have a career outside marriage.

4. Changes in legislation: it is no longer necessary to give up work with marriage and pregnancy.

Despite this, however, and the fact that in Europe only women in Denmark are more economically active:

1. Women still are concentrated in less skilled lower paid work.

2. They often fail to reach their full potential.

3. They are willing to take work of a lesser standing than that for which they are qualified.

4. They seldom reach the upper echelons of their professions.

The reasons for this are mainly:

1. Traditional Attitudes. Women are still considered a 'reserve of labour', to be called upon at times of national emergency.

2. Restrictions from Domestic Responsibilities.

3. Women's Attitudes. Success in career is in conflict with the idea of being feminine.

4. Career Conflicts. Which partner should have the dominant career? and difficulties arising where mobility is required for a particular job.

The dominant reason why women are not as successful in the employment field as men must surely be that the majority of women still marry and have children; women do not therefore have the time or energy to compete and succeed.

THE REPRODUCTIVE HAZARDS OF WOMEN AT WORK

This subject is becoming one of increasing interest with the movement of women into what has been traditional male employment, e.g. 28·4% of workers in the chemical/pharmaceutical industry are now women.

There is one fundamental difference between the sexes and that is the ability of the woman to bear children. One cannot deny that even in this respect men have an essential role to play. Until recently this aspect of human physiology was ignored when setting hygiene standards.

Factors Affecting Pregnancy

1. Physical

a. Lifting weights: ILO recommends that the maximum weight to be lifted by a woman should be *about* 50% of that for the adult male worker.

b. Working: more women now work during pregnancy and tend to work until at least 28 weeks' gestation. There has been much conflicting evidence on the effect of work on the outcome of pregnancy. In women with a long working week and in those whose work is physically tiring the proportion of pre-term (<37/52) births may be increased. Birth weight may also be affected.

c. Visual display units: no solid epidemiological evidence is available which states that VDUs present a hazard in pregnancy. However, following reports of a clustering of abnormal births to women working with VDUs in Canada in 1980, further studies are needed.

d. Ionizing radiation: ionizing radiation is both mutagenic and teratogenic. Maternal exposure to ionizing radiation may well increase the risk of the development of leukaemia in later childhood.

e. Disturbances in circadian rhythms: it has been shown that air crews with frequent time zone shifts suffer disturbances to their circadian rhythms. This is said to affect the menstrual cycle and ovarian function resulting in menstrual irregularity, most probably due to a prolongation of the pre-ovulatory phase of menstruation.

f. Shift work: the working lifestyle of an individual may well result in problems of procreation, either by interfering with normal social life or with tiredness affecting libido.

2. Biological

a. Rubella: well known to be a teratogen.

b. Cytomegalovirus: a recent review has concluded that CMV is not a serious occupational risk.

c. Viruses: a Canadian study looked at the outcome of pregnancies to nurses who had worked with children. The methodology was questionable but did show an increase in unspecified types of congenital malformations reported compared with babies of nurses so exposed. The study did not show a relationship between miscarriage and employment exposure.

3. Psychological. Stress: adrenaline is known to be an experimental teratogen and it may be that stress induces teratogenic effects.

4. Chemicals. Exposure limits are based on a 70-kg man but available evidence suggests that for airborne contaminants this is also applicable for a 50-kg woman. When considering reproductive hazards, however, it may be necessary to review these levels.

Reproductive Risks

1. Interference with Mating Drives. Loss of libido/impotence, e.g. stilboestrol and its effect on male libido.

2. Efficiency of Conception. Direct effect on the uterus and ovaries.

Indirect effect on the pituitary with release of gonadotrophins, i.e. exposure to synthetic oestrogens, carbon bisulphide, organic solvents, formaldehyde. Male workers exposed to dibromochloropropane were shown to suffer from oligo-spermia and azoospermia.

3. Risks to the Unborn Child

Teratogen. This is a substance interfering with the normal development of the fetus causing an abnormal child to be born (from the Greek word meaning monster).

Chemical mutagen. The capacity of a chemical to bring about changes in the genetic material that can be passed from one cell to its daughter cell or from one generation to the next.

There is no evidence that any case of occupational exposure has led to the birth of an abnormal child.

For reference, a woman is defined to be of *reproductive capacity* if:

a. She is under 50 years of age.

b. Has not undergone any surgery making it impossible for her to conceive.

Examples

a. Lead has been known to be a toxin for 2000 years. It was the first known reproductive hazard, acting as an abortifacient. Lead is also a teratogen.

b. Anaesthetic gases: exposure to nitrous oxide and halothane in pregnant female anaesthetists has been shown to produce a small excess risk of small-for-dates babies. The latest studies have shown no association with increased risk of abortion.

c. Laboratory work and exposure to solvents: a Swedish study has shown a slightly increased risk but no significant difference in the miscarriage rate of female workers exposed to solvents.

d. Vinyl chloride: exposure has been shown in some studies to be associated with an increased abortion rate and raised incidence of fetal malformations.

e. Organic mercury poisoning: as in the Minamata disaster in Japan. There is an increased incidence of cerebral palsy and brain damage following *in utero* exposure. Similar results were seen in 1972 in Iraq where grain for human consumption was contaminated with organic mercury.

f. 2,3,7,8-Tetrachlorodibenzodioxin: this agent is both mutagenic and teratogenic.

g. Polychlorinated biphenyl exposure results in small-for-dates babies with darkened skins and ocular discharge.

4. Late Effects. Until recently we were ignorant of these effects; prenatal exposure to a variety of substances may result in abnormalities of postnatal development and behaviour.

Examples

Methyl mercury in Japan: some prenatally exposed children, now teenagers who originally showed no signs of toxicity are now less well co-ordinated than their school fellows.

Diethylstilboestrol: prenatal exposure of female fetuses has resulted in some cases of vaginal cancer around the time of puberty.

Polychlorinated biphenyls: prenatal exposure has resulted in some cases of neurological and behavioural effects persisting in some children up to the age of 6 years.

The present rate of knowledge about the impact of work on reproductive health is similar to that concerning carcinogenesis some 10–15 years ago. Reproductive health is an extremely complex subject with a number of different processes which can be impaired and a large number of different abnormalities can be produced. It would need a massive and sustained research effort to do anything other than scratch the surface of the problem.

Some chemicals have been shown to affect the female reproductive functions and they must be carefully evaluated before a hygiene standard is applied to the workplace. In some cases where the hygiene standard needs to be markedly reduced, it may be impossible or uneconomic to reach this level and here it may be necessary to exclude women of child-bearing capacity. But the information available suggests that there are likely to be few situations in which the non-pregnant woman will be more susceptible than a man to the effects of toxic chemicals.

References

Barlow S. M. and Sullivan F. M. (1982) *Reproductive Hazards of Occupational Chemicals.* London, Academic Press.
Nicholson J. (1984) *Men and Women: How Different are They?* Oxford, Oxford University Press.

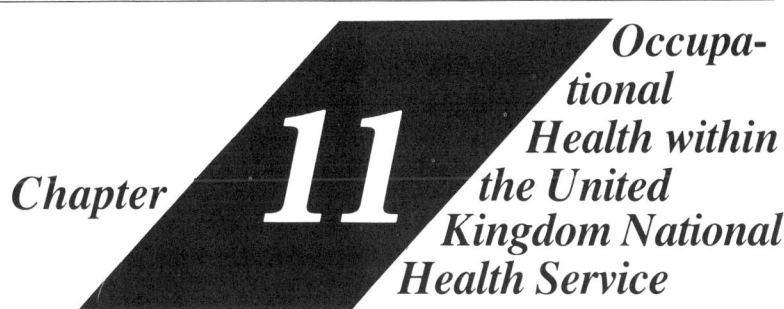

Chapter 11

Occupational Health within the United Kingdom National Health Service

HISTORY

It is a paradox that a profession which is overwhelmingly concerned with the care of others tends to neglect itself. The occupational health care of hospital staff has been at the best very patchy and arbitrary and at the worst neglected. In 1968 the Tunbridge Committee published a report, *The Care of the Health of Hospital Staff* which advocated the development of a proper service in hospitals. This report was accepted in spirit by the Government, but no additional funds were allocated and no guide-lines were issued. It is not surprising that development was slow and patchy. A few doctors and nurses were appointed, though not always did they have any specialist training or qualification. It was soon realized that these services should look at the occupational health of non-nursing staff, for example ambulance personnel, health centre staff and laundry workers.

It was not until October 1982 that the Department of Health and Social Security issued general guidance to health regions about the scope and organization of a service (Health Notice HN(82)33). Each region should identify one occupational health physician with experience and a higher qualification to advise all the districts in the region. It was later agreed that this physician should be of consultant status. The appointments were not mandatory, however, and by early 1984 only a few had been made in England and Wales, but rather more in Scotland.

FUNCTIONS

In the Health Service there are four significant differences from occupational health services in industry.

1. In each Health District there is an Accident and Emergency Department which can cope with injuries which require anything more than the simplest first aid.

2. Immunizations against infectious diseases form a major part of occupational health care.

3. Within the health service there is easy access to clinical and pathological investigations and to advice from a host of different specialists.

4. The easy flow of patients' notes throughout the hospital service presents a major problem in confidentiality of occupational health records.

SPECIFIC HAZARDS

Physical

Back injuries are more common in nurses than in women in more sedentary occupations, and they can severely limit the nurse's career. The use of mechanical aids, ergonomically designed equipment, better training and techniques should significantly reduce the hazard. The Royal College of Nursing has collaborated with the Back Pain Association in the production of a booklet *The Handling of Patients. A Guide for Nurse Managers.* (Back Pain Association, 31–33 Park Road, Teddington, TW11 0AB.)

Ergonomically designed equipment helps portering but there is still great difficulty in lifting and handling the heavy patient in bed during nursing procedures, as *Table 11.1* shows:

Table 11.1. Occupations of injured persons (% distribution) in 975 lifting accidents

Nursing Auxiliary	30
Qualified Nurse	27
Student Nurse	15
Community Nurse	6
Ambulanceman	16
Porter	3
Radiographer	0·4
Other	3

(Source: *The Lifting of Patients in the Health Service.* Health Services Advisory Committee, 1984.)

Radiation

Both ionizing and non-ionizing radiations are used in many hospital departments. Every District has its Radiological Protection Committee, which is responsible for policies and procedures, and for monitoring exposure. Hazards to staff are minimal when their guidance is followed. The highest exposure of staff to ionizing radiation occurs in radiopharmacies dispensing radioactive isotopes, but even there doses are within allowable limits. Non-ionizing radiations, such as ultraviolet, infrared, and ultrasound are used particularly in physiotherapy departments, but with built-in safeguards they create no problem. Increasingly, lasers are being used, particularly for surgery, and their development needs careful control. Other physical hazards seen from time to time include those caused by attacks from patients, and injuries from broken glassware in laboratories.

Chemical

Anxiety about anaesthetic gases, especially nitrous oxide, occurred when early retrospective surveys suggested that the chances of spontaneous abortion were doubled if pregnant women anaesthetists worked in operating theatre environment during the first trimester. A prospective survey conducted by recruiting cohorts of female doctors has now obtained information on 5428 pregnancies. There was a 2·1% reduction in birth weight in mothers working in theatres, compared to a control group of mothers working elsewhere in hospital. There was a dose-related effect; an increase in hours of maternal work in theatre was associated with a decrease in birth weight. Women working over 30 hours per week had low birth weight babies in 12·4% of pregnancies, twice the expected rate. There was a strong association between maternal smoking and miscarriage, but standardized miscarriage rates showed no constant evidence that anaesthetists had a higher risk of miscarriage than other groups. Women not working in pregnancy had the lowest rates, doctors working in theatres (not as anaesthetists) had variably increased rates and in general women working had higher rates than non-working women. There was no evidence of an increase in congenital malformations or of stillbirths in any one occupational group. During this survey it was noted that scavenging, through suitable ducting systems, occurred more frequently as DHSS recommendations came into effect. (Knill-Jones R. P. (1983) *Occupational Factors and Pregnancy outcome in Doctors*, MFCM Dissertation.)

Cytotoxic drugs, used for immunosuppression or the chemotherapy of cancer act by interfering with cell division. They can themselves be mutagenic, teratogenic and carcinogenic. Most are irritant and can be absorbed by inhalation or through the skin. Careful handling techniques are needed. There is a guidance note for the safe handling of cytotoxic drugs (HSE Guidance Note MS21 *Precautions for the Safe Handling of Cytotoxic Drugs*). Departments servicing equipment containing mercury need to have carefully detailed procedures to prevent long-term exposure. Chronic mercury poisoning has been described in dentists who have been careless in handling amalgam. Many of the chemicals encountered are irritants and some are sensitizers. Streptomycin and cytotoxic drugs are common examples. Formalin is used in the laboratories and sterile supply departments, it is a powerful irritant to skin and mucous membranes and can sometimes produce bronchospasm.

Glutaraldehyde is a disinfecting agent used particularly in the care of endoscopes. It is a highly efficient disinfectant against bacteria, spores and viruses but it is also a powerful irritant and sensitizer. It is gradually being replaced by better cleansing techniques and other less irritant but also less effective disinfectants. Asthma resulting from sensitization to mouse urine is a prescribed disease and occurs occasionally in laboratory research workers.

Biological

This is an important group of hazards in the health service. Occupational health has two distinct functions: to prevent staff from infecting patients and to protect the staff against infection.

The health surveillance must include procedures to exclude staff with active tuberculosis, catering staff with intestinal infections and to treat nursing staff working in surgical areas or where dressings are done if they suffer from any skin infections or discharges. The multi-resistant *Staphylococcus aureus* is a particular problem.

Hospital staff need to be protected against the following infections:

a. Tuberculosis. Staff with little or no response to a tuberculin test should be immunized with BCG vaccine.

b. Rubella. All female staff of child-bearing age should be tested for rubella antibodies and offered immunization, if susceptible. Male staff working in obstetric units should also be immune.

c. Cytomegalovirus. This normally causes a fairly trivial illness, but it can have disastrous effects on a fetus in the early stages of pregnancy. There is a fairly high incidence of infection amongst sick babies, but there is no evidence that they transmit the infection to staff. No vaccine is available.

d. Hepatitis 'B'. The virus is carried in the blood and tissue fluids of sufferers and carriers. Blood is the most common vector material; spread from urine and saliva is less likely. The virus is present during the prodromal and active stage of the disease and, in some cases, a chronic carrier state ensues. Occurrence of a chronic carrier state is relatively low in Europe, Australia and North America (1–5 per 1000); it is highest (5–15%) in inter-tropical Africa and in South-East Asia. It is said that certain categories of people, for example, those suffering from Down's syndrome, are high-risk carriers. It is not certain if this is specific; it seems more likely that it is because many of these people tended to be institutionalized and kept in a close community. Surveys of such communities have shown varying results. One conducted in North America demonstrated a 10–20% carrier state in institutions for the mentally retarded. Another study showed no evidence of excess morbidity due to hepatitis B in 2000 employees of an institution for the mentally retarded, over a 10-year period. The authors conclude that hepatitis B vaccination of staff was not warranted (Lohiya G., Lohiya S., Caires, Shirley *et al.* (1984) Occupational exposure to hepatitis B virus. *J. Occup. Med.* **26**, 189–196).

A study in 1982 showed prevalence of HB virus exposure and annual attack rates in representative groups. A summary of the results is given in *Table 11.2.*

Table 11.2. Annual attack rates (%) in representative groups

Health Care Workers	
Dialysis Staff	3–11
Oral Surgeons	5 (estimated)
Staff of Custodial Institutions	13–20
Surgeons	5
Nurses in High Risk Units	1–11
Laboratory Technicians	1–3
General Physicians	2 (estimated)
Surgical House Officers	4–10
General Nurses	1

(Source: Mulley A. G., Silverstein M. D. and Dienstag J. L. (1982) Indications for the use of hepatitis 'B' vaccine, based on cost-effectiveness analysis. *N. Engl. J. Med.* (1982) Sept. 644–652.)

A common means of infection is through pricking from a used needle or scalpel blade ('needle prick injuries'). Staff so accidentally injured, however trivially, should seek advice immediately. If they are not immune, passive immunization by hyperimmune gammaglobulin is advised. Recent work shows that the new vaccine for active immunization may even confer some immunity after the first injection and it may possibly be used as an alternative to gammaglobulin. Staff at special risk should be offered active immunity.

e. Anterior Poliomyelitis. This is now a rare condition, but it can arise sporadically. All staff should be immunized.

f. Tetanus. Although there is no specific risk to hospital staff, immunization should be recommended, to keep up the level of immunity throughout the population.

Other protection may be offered to groups at special risk at different times, such as infectious disease units, laboratories and postmortem room attendants. This includes typhoid, diphtheria and much more rarely, rabies. The special risks to clinical laboratory and postmortem room staffs have been well covered by a report of a working party under the chairmanship of Sir James Howie (Howie Report) published in 1978 — *Code of Practice for the Prevention of Infection in Clinical Laboratories and Post Mortem Rooms*. This classifies micro-organisms, viruses and materials, sets up safety procedures, medical surveillance, personal precautions and laboratory procedures. Guidance notes for handling dangerous pathogens, such as smallpox, rabies, lassa fever and marburg viruses, are contained in *A Guide to the Health and Safety (Dangerous Pathogens) Regulations 1981*. Health and Safety Booklet HS(R) 12.

Psychological

It is probable that those who are attracted to medicine, nursing and ancillary professions have a higher degree of sensitivity than average. That being so, they could also be more vulnerable and more easily stressed than their contemporaries. In the process of maturing in the course of training, they will need to develop the balance between compassion and firmness that marks out a good 'carer'. *Aequanimitas and Other Addresses* by Sir William Osler should be compulsory reading for the newly qualified doctor and nurse.

Because of the easy access to drugs, there is always a risk of addiction in health care workers. This should be minimized by high standards of monitoring and discipline. Those caught misusing drugs need compassionate but firm handling.

Suicide is commoner in the medical profession than in most others — largely because of the ease of access practitioners have to drugs, and their knowledge of dosages and effects. Incidence of alcoholism, too, appears to be higher than in other professions.

The management of the 'sick doctor' and also of other sick health care professionals is a thorny problem, which has not so far had a totally satisfactory solution, but it is a matter that is of great concern to the occupational physician within the Health Service. The potential of harming patients when a doctor is schizophrenic or alcoholic is horrific, and examples, fortunately rare, can be cited.

Demands, both explicit and implicit, by patients can be limitless; they have to be balanced against the professional carer's own resources. A high standard of personal commitment with skilled and sympathetic care can only be given when the

Table 11.3.   Some standardized mortality ratios
of health service workers

Occupation and Cause of Death	SMR
Doctors	
Accidental poisoning	818
Suicide	335
Cirrhosis of Liver	311
Nurses	
Diseases of musculoskeletal system	
and connective tissue	443
Suicide	297
Injury (undetermined whether accidental	
or purposeful)	341
Pharmacists	
Suicide	464

(Source: *Occupational Mortality*. Registrar-General's Decennial Supplement for England and Wales. 1970.)

carer is well (i.e. has a high standard of physical, mental and social well-being —
WHO definition of Health). This is the objective of an occupational health service
for health care staff.

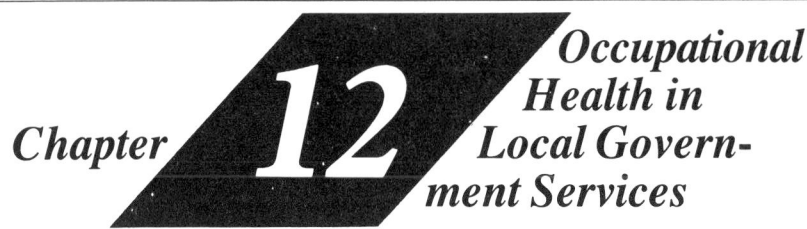
In the UK the police, fire, education, social services, highways construction and maintenance, waste disposal and some other services are all managed by local government in the rural and metropolitan counties. Before the 1974 reorganization of the Health Service local government was also responsible for some community health services, overseen by Medical Officers of Health. Some sort of rudimentary occupational health care could be offered to local government staff, but this was usually limited to the medical examination of recruits and of ill-health retirement cases. Yet there are many local services with considerable occupational health problems, the Fire Service being a notable example. After the 1974 reorganization the functions of the former Medical Officer of Health were transferred to the Health Service, and local government was left without any medical service. Now most local authorities have an occupational health service of some kind, some sharing a service with the District Health Authority, others having their own full-time service. The typical county will have approximately 40 000 employees in a wide range of occupations. They are scattered over a large geographical area, so treatment is limited to maintaining a first aid service.

SEWER MEN

Historically, we should start with this occupation as it was the observation of labourers digging out a cesspit which prompted Ramazzini to study the diseases of work. In 1832, Thackrah wrote 'With the exception of asphyxia, however, these men are not, as far as we could ascertain, subject to any serious disease, nor are they short-lived.'

The hazards are combated by good selection, training and safety standards.

Physical Hazards. Only the largest sewers are of sufficient diameter for a man to stand up. The majority of sewers are less than 6 ft in diameter; for maintenance work men have to crawl along and work, often handling heavy bricks and materials, in a confined space on a wet surface. There is a danger of being swept away or of being drowned if there is sudden flooding. On new sewer construction, particularly the deeper main sewers, the work is often done in compressed air.

Chemical Hazards. The sewer must be vented above and below the work and the atmosphere tested before the men work below. There is danger from hydrogen sulphide, methane and carbon dioxide as a result of bacterial action. There is also the danger of industrial contamination from petrol, benzene and other flammable or toxic discharges.

Biological. Sewermen are in danger of infection with any of the enteric diseases and, because of rat infestation, there is a danger of Weil's disease. Protective clothing and a good standard of personal hygiene are necessary. When men are working a long way from the depot they should have suitable portable washing facilities. Each sewer worker should have a pocket card containing notes about leptospirosis which he presents to his doctor in the event of any unusual illness.

Psychological Factors. A sewer worker must be intelligent enough to understand the dangers of his work, he has to be well disciplined in safety precautions and he must not suffer from claustrophobia.

Standards of Fitness. The man with the long thin back is particularly vulnerable to back problems when he has to work so much in a crouched position. Sewer men must have no cardiovascular disease, should have good lung function, no limb disability, good vision with full visual fields, good speech and hearing and no history of epilepsy. There are no statutory requirements for medical standards or periodic medical examinations. However, it is sensible to apply a medical selection to the recruit and although periodic examinations are not mandatory, sewer workers and their management often request them.

FIRE BRIGADES

Each county has its fire brigade, which is autonomous, but recruitment, training and some of the more advanced training facilities are shared. The Home Office sets down certain rules and codes, one of which contains the medical standards for recruitment. Fire-fighting is an extremely hazardous occupation. The mandatory requirements and medical surveillance are rudimentary and only in the last few years has there been much interest in the occupational health of firemen. At present there is no requirement for a medical examination after the age of recruitment (usually 18 to 20 years) until the fireman reaches the age of 40; then he is invited to attend a medical examination every three years. This means that the young fireman has no medical supervision during the most active part of his career. Most branches of the Fire Brigades Union have now requested and obtained much improved medical surveillance on a voluntary basis.

The Home Office has sponsored two large research projects, *A Study of Causes of Death in Firemen*, Research Report No. 20; and *Health Monitoring Scheme for Firemen*, Research Report No. 16. These will be referred to later.

Physical Hazards. The fireman has to work in an environment which is entirely outside his control. There may be extremes of heat and humidity which will stretch his physical endurance to the limit. His protective clothing and breathing apparatus add to his physical burden and, in addition, he may have to lift and carry casualties through débris or down ladders with safety. The Home Office standards of fitness for recruitment are rudimentary and examine only the man's static fitness, i.e. the absence of physical disease or deformity. More brigades are now carrying out exercise tolerance tests to ensure that recruits have a good standard of athletic fitness.

A high standard of training and discipline reduces accidents to a minimum and figures show a reasonable comparison with some other industries (*Table 12.1*).

Table 12.1.   Industrial accidents

	Non-fatal (per 1000 at risk)	*Fatal* (per 100 000 at risk)
Metal manufacture	78·9	13·5
Shipbuilding	72·4	12·8
Fire Service	63·2	16·7
Construction industry	38·4	19·9
Textile industry	26·8	1·6

Training is so important that there are more non-fatal accidents during drill, training and station duties than there are on fire-fighting (*Tables 12.2, 12.3*).

Table 12.2.   Accidents in Cheshire County Fire Service 1977–1978

On operational duties	26·7%
On drill, training and station duties	73·3%

Table 12.3.   Causes of accidents on duty

Circumstances	*Number of accidents*	*% of total*
Lifting, handling equipment/debris	14	27·5
Falls and slips	14	27·5
Hit by falling debris	9	17·6
Cuts, knocks and bruises	7	13·7
Affected by toxic fumes	3	5·8
Burnt by fire or hot object	2	3·9
Miscellaneous	2	3·9
	51	

Burns do not feature high on the list of causes of accidents. Whilst the number of fatal injuries (firemen and civilian victims) due to burns has remained almost constant, the number of fatalities due to toxic fumes has quadrupled in the last 30 years, which is most likely due to the more widespread use of plastic materials.

Chemical Hazards. There are two main sources of chemical hazard to firemen. Any large spillage, for example from a damaged road tanker, is dealt with by firemen. Fire Brigades in industrial areas have chemical incident units where the men can wear full protective clothing and can go through a thorough decontamination drill before coming off duty.

The other, and more sinister, danger is from fumes and smoke from fires. The effects of thermal degradation can be summarized as follows:

1. O_2 depletion.
2. CO_2 excess leading to hyperventilation.
3. CO formation in large quantities.
4. SO_2 causing respiratory irritation, oedema and asphyxia.
5. HCN (an endothermic reaction) formed at higher temperatures, marked increase above 700 °C. Lethal quantities even when fumes are diluted with air.
6. HCl (from PVC).

ppm	Symptoms
1–5	Limit of odour
5–10	Mild irritation of mucous membranes
35	Irritation of throat
50–100	Barely tolerable
1000	Lung oedema after short exposure

7. Aliphatic hydrocarbons: Thermal degradation of all organic polymers releases aliphatic hydrocarbons; acids; alcohols and aldehydes, including acrolein, formaldehyde, acetaldehyde, and butaldehyde. Acrolein is very irritant, extreme lacrimatory effect. MAC 0·1 ppm.

Some Known Hazards

Carbon Monoxide. This is present in all fires, but especially plastics. Even after dilution with air the level of CO may cause severe poisoning.

Plastics. PVC: Will liberate large quantities of HCl fume. *Polyurethane:* Will form HCN in lethal quantities even after dilution with fresh air. Aliphatic and aromatic hydrocarbons are also formed, but any toxic effects are greatly overshadowed by CO and HCl or HCN.

Isocyanates. (Compounds containing one or more — N=C=O groups)

i. *Bulk isocyanates:* The isocyanates are intensely irritant. 0·1 part per million of vapour is detected by smell and is potentially harmful. Exposure to isocyanate vapour causes intense irritation of the eyes, nose and throat, tightness of the chest, leading to acute bronchospasm, gross airways obstruction and respiratory distress.

ii. *Isocyanates contained in other products:* Isocyanates are used in the production of polyurethane and have a wide application: rigid foam resins, synthetic rubber, plastic coating of wire, paints, varnishes, lacquers, adhesives, etc. Some free isocyanate may be liberated by burning of these materials. Symptoms may be delayed for several hours.

Fertilizers. Most artificial fertilizers contain nitrogen, often in the form of ammonium nitrate. Burning will cause the evolution of thick brown nitrous fumes. Oxides of nitrogen are intense respiratory irritants. Only slight irritation is felt at the time of exposure; pulmonary oedema (potentially fatal) occurs up to 48 hours later.

Summary

Immediate systemic effects. CO; HCN
Immediate irritant effects. HCl; Isocyanates; Ammonia; Oxides of nitrogen.

Delayed effects. Isocyanates: obstructive airways disease. Oxides of nitrogen: potentially fatal pulmonary oedema.

It is very difficult to predict what products might occur as there are so many variables including the temperature, amount of oxygen available, presence of water, presence of additives in the form of plasticisers, antioxidants, foaming agents, stabilizers, pigments and fire retardants. There is some evidence (in animal experiments only) that some fire retardants give combustion products which can cause convulsions.

Firemen who believe they are being affected by toxic fumes are taken to the nearest accident and emergency unit. It is important that the casualty staff have some knowledge of fire hazards, otherwise the fireman who may appear to be reasonably fit may be discharged, only to suffer from intense pulmonary oedema some hours later.

Respiratory Disease in Firemen. In 1974 Peters et al. published a Study of Respiratory Function in Boston Fire Fighters in the *New England Journal of Medicine*. They found that over a two-year period firemen experienced a greater than twofold drop in the expected rate of loss of lung function and that this correlated with fire exposure. In 1976 Axford et al. (*British Journal of Industrial Medicine*) reported on an accidental exposure to isocyanate fumes when 35 men were exposed to toluene di-isocyanate. Four years later 20 had persistent respiratory symptoms but there had been a marked decline in respiratory function for the first six months only, then the trend was reversed. In 1976 Lequesne et al. (*British Journal of Industrial Medicine*) reported on persistent neurological complications in the same group of men. In 1980 Unger (*Thorax*) reported on severe smoke exposure in 30 Texas firemen; he found a decrement in FEC and FEV_1:FEC ratio, compared with matched controls.

The Home Office Research Report No. 16 *Health Monitoring Scheme for Firemen* was published in 1980. This was a longitudinal study of a sample of firemen from the London Fire Brigade. They submitted an MRC respiratory questionnaire and had their FVC and FEV_1 measured, the tests being repeated one year later. The results showed a strong negative effect of cigarette smoking on all measures of lung function. There was evidence of a more rapid fall in FEV_1 and FEC in those aged over 40. There was no demonstrable effect of length of service on pulmonary function except possibly in men with over 20 years' service. This fits in with most of the impressions of the fire brigade doctors in the UK; respiratory disease is not a specific hazard to firemen in the UK because the men are highly trained and disciplined to wear breathing apparatus whenever toxic fumes are suspected, in contrast to the practice of over 20 years ago, when a fireman thought breathing apparatus should be used very much as the last resort and firemen had to learn to 'eat smoke'.

Biological Hazards. In addition to fire-fighting, firemen are also trained in rescue work and they have special lifting and cutting equipment to release casualties trapped in road and rail accidents. They are required to do some rather dirty and obnoxious work in retrieving dead bodies; they also supervise the destruction of animals by fire when there is an outbreak of anthrax. It is important that their tetanus immunization is kept up to date and that they have appropriate medical surveillance if they are exposed to any other biological hazards.

Psychological. The presence of claustrophobia is an obvious indication against recruitment into the fire service. However, a few of the older and more experienced men develop claustrophobia and have to be medically retired. This is probably a symptom of general stress after many years of working where there are intense physical and psychological stresses. A fireman has to be able to become immediately alert when responding to an alarm and the fire services maintain a standard of discipline and drill which is at least as good as that in the Armed Forces. A fireman has to withstand the psychological shock of retrieving burnt and mutilated bodies.

The need for an immediate alert response to an alarm has suggested that there may be an increased risk of ischaemic heart disease in fire-fighters. In 1959 Mastromatteo studied 26 000 man years of experience of fire-fighters in Toronto from 1921 to 1953, and found a highly significant excess of deaths from cardiovascular-renal disease. He pointed to overweight and lack of regular physical activity as possible explanations, together with strain on the cardiovascular system related to the occupation; he thought these factors were probably aggravating rather than causal. The 1971 census in England and Wales showed that in firemen, disease of the circulatory system showed a 4% decrease, but there was a 10% excess for ischaemic heart disease. It is difficult to draw conclusions, especially because of the 'healthy worker effect'. It is likely that the position will change during the next few years as the standard of fitness required in recruitment is now much higher and there is much more emphasis on the maintaining of physical fitness during service. Many brigades have now introduced fitness programmes, and overweight and cigarette smoking are discouraged.

The Home Office Research Report No. 20 *A Study of Causes of Death in Firemen* is inconclusive but shows the need for a more detailed and widespread study. Of the brigades studied, some showed a decrease and some an increase in deaths from ischaemic heart disease. However, it does seem probable that there is a small increased risk of ischaemic heart disease, together with a decrease for all causes of death combined. There is no evidence of any increased risk from respiratory disease.

POLICEMEN

Modern police administration in Great Britain began in 1829 with the establishment of the Metropolitan Police. Constabularies in some of the counties began about 1840 and gradually the smaller borough constabularies amalgamated into larger police forces with a single Chief Constable in charge. The police forces are responsible to local police committees but central government, through the Home Secretary, maintains a certain degree of surveillance through Inspectors of Constabulary and introduces some degree of co-ordination into a system which is almost wholly decentralized. There are major political arguments concerning the advantages and disadvantages of a centrally organised police force under Government control.

Physical Hazards
Figures given in *Table 12.4* show the trend for injuries on duty and injuries due to assault during the past six years.

Table 12.4. Cheshire constabulary. Injuries causing absence from duty per 1000 police men and women

Year	On duty excluding assault		Due to assault	
	Number of Injuries	Days off Sick	Number of Injuries	Days off Sick
1978	40	827	8·5	280
1983	60	1388	26	834

Noise-induced deafness may be caused by firearm drill, particularly if it takes place in a confined space. For radiotelephone communication police motor-cyclists have earphones within their helmets. Investigations of the ambient noise created by wind flow in these helmets showed that the daily noise dose measured lay closely around the recommended limit. It is recommended that every police officer who is to carry out motor-cyclist duties undergoes an audiometric test before starting and thereafter at annual intervals. So far monitoring has failed to show any significant hearing loss.

A number of forces have underwater search units, where the men are medically supervised for using underwater breathing apparatus.

Chemical Hazards. Some firearm instructors working in indoor ranges were found to have high blood lead concentrations. A certain amount of lead is dispersed into the atmosphere when each bullet is fired. Suitable ventilation of indoor ranges adequately deals with the problem.

Scenes of crime officers use a fine aluminium powder to dust over surfaces to reveal finger prints. There was concern that officers working in a confined space might inhale a large quantity of aluminium powder. This led some constabularies to arrange an annual chest X-ray for all officers exposed. However, this would seem to be unnecessary as investigation done by the TUC Centenary Institute of Occupational Health showed that although concentrations of aluminium powder varied considerably, according to the technique used, all were well below the threshold limit value. Nevertheless, officers are advised to avoid excessive use of the powder, especially in confined spaces.

CS smoke may be used for dealing with armed criminals, but its use is very rare. It is highly irritant, causing a burning sensation in the eyes with intense lacrimation, irritation of the respiratory tract with sneezing, tightness in the chest, dyspnoea and cough. High concentrations may cause nausea and vomiting. It irritates exposed skin, especially if it is moist. Washing, fresh air and eye irrigation are usually the only treatments required.

Biological Hazards. In dealing with drug addicts policemen may be exposed to infection by hepatitis B virus. They should be offered the same protection as health care workers and any soiled clothing should be replaced. Tetanus immunity should be maintained and protection against rabies offered when necessary.

Psychological Hazards. There are a number of psychological stresses, some of which are peculiar to police work. Most police officers have to work on a shift rota. Many young policemen marry policewomen, and although wherever possible it is arranged for them both to be on the same shift, shift work creates difficulties in family and social life.

Perhaps the most important and most difficult stress arises from the police officer's duty to uphold the law and his vulnerability to criticism. Early in his career he has to learn to cope with aggressive interrogation when he appears in court. He also has to respond to violence without being violent himself. He may be the victim of a great deal of verbal abuse, and at times severe physical abuse but he has to resist the temptation, and the natural reflex, to strike back. Simulated court appearances and riot conditions are now provided in his early training programme.

Medical Standards for Recruitment. Obviously the recruit must be physically and mentally fit. There is no need to itemize each test, but most constabularies insist on a minimum height of 5ft 8in for a man or 5ft 4in for a woman. Whilst the accepted standard of vision is 6/6 in each eye, which may be corrected provided the uncorrected vision is not worse than 6/18 in each eye, it is now generally recognized that it is better to recruit people with good vision who need no glasses. As with the firemen, it is important to assess the candidates' athletic fitness. Both this and mental alertness and temperament are best assessed in a practical test. A number of constabularies now use an outward bound type of course with initiative tests and quite severe tests of physical stamina. These tests substantially reduce recruit failure.

Medical Surveillance. This is limited to medical examination after sickness or injury. One constabulary conducted a pilot study on fitness and the benefits of a fitness training programme. It showed that a number of officers had a poor level of fitness which could be easily improved. Formal fitness training programmes are difficult to introduce because of shift work and frequent calls for extra duties. Nevertheless, the need for a high standard of physical fitness has been demonstrated adequately by recent events, particularly riots and picketing. Although it has not been possible to implement a fitness training programme the standard of physical fitness is improving with more awareness, example and leadership by senior officers, with better recruit selection and with riot training.

OTHER LOCAL GOVERNMENT STAFF

There are many other occupations in local government where occupational health surveillance is needed. Most of these occupations also occur in other forms of employment, but there are two which are almost unique to local government: teachers and non-medical care staff.

Teachers

It is difficult to say if there is more mental illness in teachers than in others, as estimates of mental illness in the general population vary considerably. It is certain that mental illness in teachers is a very great problem because of the nature of the work. It is not too difficult to employ some one with neurotic symptoms, or even with a well controlled psychotic illness, in a fairly large working group. The teacher, in contrast, stands alone in front of a class of children who are very perceptive and who can be incredibly unkind. As with any employee with a mental illness there tends to be a lack of understanding and fear amongst other members of the working group; this is particularly noticeable in teachers. The mentally ill teacher is not wanted in the school by the children, the other teachers, the parents or the school governors.

In 1982 Doctor Hamblett reported on a study of mental health in the teaching profession in the County Education Authority of Avon. He studied the reasons for referral of employees for an occupational health opinion; he compared 100 referred teachers, a group of 400 referred non-professional employees and a group of 175 mixed professional employees of the Council. The results are shown in *Table 12.5*

Table 12.5.   Type of illness as a percentage of referrals

	Teachers	Non-professional	Mixed professional
Physical illness	19	62	76
Neurotic illness	53	30	19
Psychotic illness	19	2·5	2·5
Other mental illness (personality disorders, etc.)	9	5	2·5

Both neurotic and psychotic illnesses present more commonly in teachers than in any other groups. It was interesting to find that in the mixed professional group there was more work-related stress than domestic stress, but in teachers the reverse was the case.

Attempts to reduce mental illness in the teaching profession should be directed to more careful selection, counselling during training, early referral for advice and arrangements for special leave or redeployment. Such preventive measures are more likely to succeed when the stigma and fear of mental illness are overcome.

Care Staff

Traditionally, old people, orphans and children who needed special care were cared for in institutions overseen by the Medical Officer of Health in each local authority; but it seemed inappropriate to have a hospital or institutionalized setting for people who really needed homes and not institutional care. The Seebohm Report (1968) sought to remedy this and the 1970 Local Authority Social Services Act facilitated the change. The special classes of people who need care in the community are now cared for by non-medical care staff in 'homes'. Elderly persons who can no longer care for themselves in their own home can be moved into an Elderly Persons' Home where there may be 20 or 30 residents, each one with his own bedroom but where there is a communal rest room and dining room. The children are cared for in homes of small numbers where the care staff try to adopt the role of parent. More recently, there have been some profound changes which have affected these original concepts.

The number of old people is greatly increasing year by year. Consequently, the hospital geriatric units can no longer cope with all the old people who need hospital care. This means that there is a tendency for many old people in elderly persons' homes to need more than just a home atmosphere; many of them are disturbed or disabled and some are quite ill. (This increases the waiting lists for the elderly persons' homes and puts an increasing burden on relatives or community care staff in attempting to care for the old people who have had to remain at home, although they are unable to care for themselves adequately.) The homes and the training of the care staff were designed to cope with the sort of residents that they were having some 14 years ago. They are finding it increasingly difficult to deal with the larger numbers of psychogeriatric or physically ill old people. Manpower reductions in local government mean that manning levels are at the absolute minimum; sickness absences in staff are covered by the other staff working longer hours; sometimes a care assistant or an officer-in-charge (matron) may work 80 hours a week. The work is extremely demanding both physically and emotionally. A number of care staff become physically exhausted and seek early retirement on medical grounds. Back injuries result from the physical demands of the job; alcoholism sometimes results from the emotional stresses and overwork.

There is a reverse trend in the children's homes; there being fewer children, adoption and fostering are easier and some children's homes are closing. However, there remain a number of children who need either short-term or long-term care because of behavioural problems and the care staff have to be emotionally stable and well-trained. There is a tendency for applicants for child care work to say 'I have many problems of my own, so I am sure I can help these poor children'. This, of course, is just the wrong sort of person to appoint. The child care officer must be emotionally very robust and it is best that he has some engrossing outside activity, otherwise it is easy for him to become too emotionally involved with the children, consequently failing to help them. There have been a number of mental health breakdowns in child care staff due to poor selection. Most employing authorities still insist on a physical examination for new employees, yet very few require any kind of examination of mental health.

There is a small and special group of teachers and care staff who look after physically disabled and educationally subnormal children, either in schools, day centres, or residential homes. Careful selection for physical and mental fitness is required; the children are very demanding in their needs and many of them require physical help in lifting and carrying. Infectious diseases, particularly the enteric infections, spread rapidly where low intelligence impairs personal hygiene. These teachers and care staff are frequently exposed to outbreaks of hepatitis A and they also need to be aware of any child who is a hepatitis B carrier.

Chapter 13

Toxicology I. General Principles

Toxicology is the study of the potential of chemicals to produce adverse effects in living organisms. It investigates their nature, the likelihood of their occurring, their detection, the means by which they are produced and how they can be prevented or reversed. Such studies are of obvious importance in relation to occupational medicine and hygiene. The aims are to define likely adverse consequences to man following exposure, to advise on the best ways to reduce or prevent the likelihood of adverse effects occurring, to plan the most appropriate methods for monitoring personnel, to detect early toxic effects and to treat accidental poisoning.

Toxic compounds may produce effects at the site of contamination (e.g. skin, eye and respiratory tract) or may be absorbed into the circulation and produce effects on specific target organs (e.g. liver, kidney) or more generally (e.g. carbon monoxide and cyanides). Chemicals which produce toxic effects following absorption may themselves be directly toxic or be converted to toxic products after metabolism. However, many substances are either excreted or converted to less toxic compounds by various metabolic processes (detoxification). In general, the adverse sequelae which may result from effects at the site of contamination are less life-threatening than those that may occur following absorption in to the circulation.

Sites of Contamination and Absorption

1. Respiratory Tract. This is the commonest route of absorption, since many toxic industrial chemicals become atmospheric pollutants. The depth to which solid materials penetrate the respiratory tract depends on the size of the particles, e.g. particles 1 μm or less usually reach the alveoli, but particles in excess of 30 μm may not enter the respiratory tract. Some inhaled toxic chemicals exert their effects locally, e.g. silicosis, pleural mesothelioma from asbestos dusts, inflammation of the upper respiratory tract by phosphorus pentoxide and titanium tetrachloride smokes, or delayed pulmonary oedema following alveolar damage by phosgene or hydrogen chloride gas. Other substances may be absorbed across the respiratory tract and exert their effects at other sites, e.g. carbon monoxide, organophosphates and organic solvents.

2. Skin. Local effects on skin may include dermatitis, corrosion and sensitization. Other chemicals may also be absorbed across the skin and produce systemic effects. A variety of factors influence the rate at which materials may be absorbed across the skin; these include molecular weight, lipid solubility, formulation of the material and the integrity of the skin.

3. Ingestion. The dust collecting in the mucus of the upper respiratory tract may be swallowed, or food and drink may become contaminated. Industrial poisoning by this route is rare.

4. Injection. Rare in industry, but examples are: (*a*) accidental injection by high pressure hydraulic systems; (*b*) injury where plutonium may be directly absorbed into the tissues. A dose in excess of the total body burden may easily be absorbed.

5. Eye. Some chemicals may produce variable degrees of eye damage following local contamination. Less frequently, a few chemicals may be absorbed across the eye or conjunctival blood vessels to produce local effects on the eye (e.g. miosis with organophosphates) or more general effects (e.g. anticholinesterase effects with potent organophosphates, or cyanide poisoning following splash contamination of the eye with concentrated solutions of hydrogen cyanide, and its alkali salts).

Fate of Toxins

1. Metabolism to non-toxic end products.
2. Metabolism to a toxic product, e.g. methanol → formaldehyde.
3. Tissue localization

> *3.1 Protein.* Some foreign substances, e.g. mercury, chromates, become bound to proteins in tissues or blood. If the binding is reversible an equilibrium is established between bound and unbound toxin. Firm binding will reduce the rate of excretion. Some toxins may act as carcinogens by becoming bound to DNA directly or indirectly after metabolism.

> *3.2 Fat.* Some compounds have a high lipid solubility and become localized in a fat tissue, e.g. DDT.

> *3.3 Bone.* Lead, strontium, and many other radioactive isotopes have an affinity for bone.

4. Sometimes there is a combination of fates, e.g. lead; some is stored, some is metabolized, and some is excreted unchanged.

Excretion of Toxins

1. A variable fraction of a volatile toxin is excreted in expired air.
2. Some toxins are excreted from the alimentary canal, either directly, or through bile after absorption into the hepatic circulation.
3. Some toxins, or their metabolites, are excreted in the urine.
4. Some toxic chemicals are excreted in the saliva. Lead is an important example.

Factors Influencing Toxic Effects

1. Quantity or concentration.

2. Duration of exposure.

3. Phase: Whether presented as solid, liquid or dispersed in the atmosphere. With solutions, for example, the degree of percutaneous absorption may depend on the formulation of the material (e.g. dimethylsulphoxide may enhance toxicity by facilitating absorption across the skin). In the atmosphere, the depth of penetration into the respiratory tract will depend upon whether the material exists as a gas or vapour, or, if in particulate form, the size of particles.

4. Tissue affinity and solubility in tissues, e.g. sulphydryl molecule, for which certain toxic agents have an affinity.

5. Sensitivity of certain tissues or organs.

6. Individual susceptibility.

Individual Susceptibility

People in the same environment, exposed to the same agent, may have differing responses. Some known factors are: previous or coexisting disease; diet (especially alcohol); constitution (fat or thin); age; sex; genetic background; fatigue; endocrine status.

Absorption and Poisoning

Absorption may take place without poisoning. Poisoning presupposes absorption. Some demonstrable biochemical effects may be found before symptoms of overt poisoning appear. The greater the knowledge of the biochemical effects, and the more sensitive the tests, the earlier they can be detected, e.g.

Lead. Raised blood lead, urinary coproporphyrin and ALA precede signs of poisoning.

Organophosphorus. Lowered red cell cholinesterase — and lowered EMG voltage.

TNT. Webster's Test indicates absorption, not poisoning.
Presence of metabolites in urine — mandelic acid from styrene, hippuric acid from toluene, phenol from benzene, trichloracetic acid from trichlorethylene — indicative of *exposure*.

Levels of Toxin in the Blood

The presence of a toxin, or its characteristic metabolite in the blood demonstrates absorption. It is a qualitative test, but the blood level is not necessarily an indicator of quantity. Soon after absorption the blood level may be high; it will decline if the toxin is stored in body tissues, and will rise again when it is mobilized. A low blood level does not necessarily mean a low total absorption dosage.

Errors in Laboratory Samples

Any single type of observation is only part of the total picture. If laboratory results do not fit with other observations, the laboratory results should be questioned first. Errors may occur in collection, accidental contamination, deterioration of the sample, technique, calculation, the mixing of specimens and in reporting. One should also question how 'normal values' are established. They may need to be modified in the light of experience.

Acute and Chronic Effects

Toxic agents may behave differently in acute and chronic poisoning, e.g. some hydrocarbons are acute narcotic agents, and they also have specific chronic effects on the liver, kidneys or nerve tissues.

Synergism

By blocking a metabolic pathway, one toxin may reduce the effective metabolism of another, and therefore enhance its toxic effects. (*See* Conjugation *below*.)

Detoxification Mechanisms

The liver is the main organ for detoxification. Most of the enzymes occur in the endoplasmic reticulum of the liver cells. Other sites include plasma and the alimentary canal.

There are two types of reaction: metabolic transformation and conjugation. Many foreign compounds are metabolized by both types of reaction.

Metabolic Transformation. The substance may be subjected to a chain of reactions including oxidation (addition of O, or subtraction of H), hydroxylation or reduction, e.g.

1. Oxidation:

$$CH_3OH \quad \rightarrow \quad HCOH \quad \rightarrow \quad HCOOH$$

Methanol   Formaldehyde   Formic acid
           (toxic)   (toxic)

2. Hydroxylation:

Benzene   Phenol

Conjugation. Some foreign compounds, or their metabolites, are combined with endogenous substances to form conjugates. The common endogenous substances used for conjugation are glucuronic acid, glycine, sulphate, acetyl and methyl groups. They add on to a reactive group of the toxin, e.g. hydroxyl, amino, carboxyl, halogen, epoxide. The endogenous conjugation substrates are polarized, thus increasing water solubility and aiding renal excretion, e.g.

1. Benzene will be metabolized to phenol, which may then be conjugated with glucuronic acid and sulphate, giving phenol glucuronide and phenol sulphate. The

presence of urinary sulphate of benzene is a demonstration of benzene absorption. If a mixture of carbon tetrachloride and benzene is absorbed, the CCl_4 will affect the liver and may interfere with benzene conjugation. This is an example of synergism (*see above*).

2. Glycine conjugation: results in the secretion of hippuric acid, e.g.

Toluene   Hippuric acid

There are many other reactions of metabolism and conjugation, e.g. deamination, de-chlorination, de-hydroxylation, acetylation. Often a combination of mechanisms takes place.

Threshold Limit Values (TLV)

Some potentially toxic chemicals appear naturally in our environment, e.g. heavy metals present in soil may appear in food, and pesticide residues may also be ingested with food. The ingestion of some chemicals is controlled by recommended acceptable daily intake (ADIs). In the industrial setting it may not be practical or even possible to achieve zero environmental exposure to a given toxic chemical. It thus follows that industry needs some levels of occupational hygiene standard, at least as a guide to where first to aim. For inhalation hazards the TLV is currently used.

The TLV is intended to represent the level, at or below which it is unlikely that impairment of health will occur in a normal person if the exposure lasts for normal working hours during a normal working lifetime. The TLV is the *currently accepted* standard; it cannot be regarded as an acknowledged and permanent standard. For example, the TLV for benzene has been reduced progressively from 100 to 5 ppm. The TLV is not an upper limit of safety; some susceptible individuals may be affected below this level. The theoretical conversion of a TLV to a Lethal Concentration 50 would show that it represents a level of dosage between 1/10th and 1/1000th of the LC_{50}.

TLVs are standards accepted by the American Conference of Government Industrial Hygienists. The list is published annually after a study of all the available literature. Some recommendations and alterations are based on industrial and epidemiological experience, and in some cases on controlled human volunteer observations, e.g. the TLV for methylene chloride has been lowered on the basis of observations in man which show this substance to be metabolized to carbon monoxide, leading to increases in carboxyhaemoglobin levels. Many values are obtained as a result of animal experiments; sometimes a value is adopted on flimsy evidence which may be all that is available at the time. In the absence of any new scientific data the TLV is a useful guide, as it is based on a review of current knowledge. At the moment there are TLVs for only about 5% of the marketed chemicals.

In the United Kingdom the Health and Safety Executive has now produced its own list of Control Limits for toxic materials (*see* p. 117). Control Limits apply to a limited list of substances which are the subject of Regulations, Codes of Practice or EEC directives. For other materials, there are Recommended Limits which are those advised by the Advisory Committee on Toxic Substances of the Health and Safety Commission. With few exceptions, these limits are identical with the TLVs listed by the American Conference of Government Industrial Hygienists (ACGIH), and in Chapter 14 TLVs are still shown as such, except where a British Control Limit has been established.

Time-weighted Average (TWA) Limits

With some substances exposure above the TLV may be permitted for short periods, if this is compensated by equivalent periods below the TLV, provided there are no cumulative effects and the acute toxicity level is not reached. The excursion TLV factor defines the magnitude of the permissible excursion above the limit.

For some other substances there is a very small margin between TLV and the level where irritation or toxic effects will appear. For these substances the TLV must be regarded as a ceiling value, i.e. a maximal allowable concentration (MAC).

OCCUPATIONAL EXPOSURE LIMITS

(Guidance Note EH 40 from the Health and Safety Executive)

Introduction

1. This Guidance Note gives advice on limits to which exposure to airborne substances hazardous to health should be controlled in workplaces. These limits form part of the criteria which are used by the Health and Safety Executive (HSE) in assessing compliance with the Health and Safety at Work etc Act 1974 (HSW Act) and other relevant statutory provisions.

2. It lists the following occupational exposure limits, viz. control limits and recommended limits, but it does not contain limits for chemical substances which are hazardous solely on account of their radioactive properties.

3. It replaces Guidance Note EH 15/80 and will be reprinted annually with any necessary revisions.

Legal Requirements

4. Section 2 of the HSW Act places upon employers a duty to ensure, so far as is reasonably practicable, the health, safety and welfare at work of all their employees. Employers and the self-employed are required by Section 3 to conduct their undertakings in such a way as to ensure, so far as is reasonably practicable, that persons not in their employment who may be affected by these work activities are not thereby exposed to risks to their health and safety.

5. Section 6 requires manufacturers, importers and suppliers of substances for use at work to ensure, so far as is reasonably practicable, that the substances are safe and without risks to health when properly used. It also requires these persons to carry out such testing and examination as may be necessary and to secure that

adequate information will be available about the results of any relevant tests which have been carried out in connection with the substances and about any conditions necessary to ensure that they will be safe and without risks to health when properly used.

6. More specific requirements relating to particular processes and substances and places of work are contained in other relevant statutory provisions which include the Factories Act 1961, the Mines and Quarries Act 1954, the Agriculture (Poisonous Substances) Act 1952 and regulations made under these Acts or under the HSW Act.

Interpretation

7. Whilst only the Courts can give a binding decision on the interpretation of these legal requirements, some practical guidance can be given. There are two key phrases in the requirements of the HSW Act; first 'to ensure, … the health, safety and welfare at work … ' and second, 'so far as is reasonably practicable'.

8. The first phrase sets the objective to be achieved. The method of achieving it is largely left to the person on whom the duty is placed although he must pay heed to any more specific requirements which amplify the general duties. In terms of preventing ill-health from exposure to substances hazardous to health, these obligations are usually met by eliminating or minimising exposure to such substances.

9. The duty to ensure health and safety at work in the HSW Act is qualified by the phrase 'so far as is reasonably practicable'. Although this expression is not defined in the Act, it has acquired quite a clear meaning through long established interpretations by the Courts. Someone who is required to do something 'so far as is reasonably practicable' must assess, on the one hand, the magnitude of the risks of a particular work activity or environment, and, on the other hand, the physical difficulty, time, trouble and expense which would be involved in taking steps to eliminate or minimise those risks. If, for example, the risks to health and safety of a particular work process are very low, and the cost or technical difficulties of taking certain steps to avoid those risks are very high, it might not be reasonably practicable to take those steps. The greater the degree of risk, the less weight can be given to the cost of measures needed to avoid that risk. Only if there is a gross disproportion between them, the reduction in risk being insignificant in relation to the sacrifices needed to achieve the reduction, is the obligation met.

10. The comparison does not include the financial standing of the employer. A precaution which is 'reasonably practicable' for a prosperous employer is equally 'reasonably practicable' for the less affluent. Furthermore, if someone is prosecuted for failing to comply with a duty 'so far as is reasonably practicable', it is the responsibility of the accused to show the court that it was not reasonably practicable for him to do more than he had in fact done to comply with the duty.

Control of Exposure

11. Exposure to substances can result in intake into the body by inhalation, ingestion or absorption through the skin or by a combination of these. Inhalation is usually the most important route of entry into the body.

12. Exposure should be kept as low as is reasonably practicable, primarily by the application of suitable material, plant and process control techniques. The use of personal protective equipment should be considered as a method of protection

only in those situations where the risks cannot be controlled at source, rather than as a first line of defence. In certain cases, notably during maintenance, plant emergencies or non-routine work, personal protection may be the only reasonably practicable measure. In these cases, care must also be taken to avoid exposure of others who may be in the vicinity and are unprotected.

Health Surveillance

13. Health surveillance of workers is often an important concomitant to environmental control. Guidance Note MS 20[1] describes the circumstances in which pre-employment health screening or medical examination may make a useful contribution to occupational health care and gives guidance on the conduct of screening and examinations. General principles on which routine health surveillance of employed persons at work may be undertaken are set out in Guidance Note MS 18[2] for the use of employers and others concerned with the prevention of occupational illness and disease.

Occupational Exposure Limits

14. The list of occupational exposure limits given in this Guidance Note relates to personal exposure (*see* paragraph 25) and is divided into two parts.

Part 1: Control Limits

15. Part 1 lists those exposure limits which are contained in Regulations, Approved Codes of Practice, in European Community Directives or which have been adopted by the Health and Safety Commission (HSC). They are limits which have been judged after detailed consideration of the available scientific and medical evidence to be 'reasonably practicable' for the whole spectrum of work activities in Great Britain. These exposure limits are known specifically as control limits and should not normally be exceeded.

16. Further action may be necessary to fulfil the requirements of the HSW Act even when the control limit is observed. This is most likely to occur with substances for which there are no apparent thresholds below which adverse effects do not occur or where exposure to relatively high concentrations over very short periods may be injurious. In such cases, not only should exposure not exceed the control limits given in Part 1 of the list, but exposure should also be reduced still further until the point is reached where the costs of further control measures are not justified in terms of the additional reduction in risk.

17. The Health and Safety Executive will use control limits in determining whether, in their opinion, the requirements of the relevant legislation are being observed. Failure to comply with control limits, or to reduce exposure still further, where this is reasonably practicable, may result in enforcement action.

Part 2: Recommended Limits

18. Exposure limits recommended by the Health and Safety Executive on advice from HSC's Advisory Committee on Toxic Substances (ACTS) are listed in Part 2. These limits are considered to represent good practice and realistic criteria for the control of exposure, plant design, engineering controls and, if necessary, the selection and use of personal protective equipment. Health and Safety Executive inspectors will use these exposure limits as part of their criteria

for assessing compliance with the HSW Act and other relevant statutory provisions.

19. The further action noted in paragraph 16 relating to substances for which there is no apparent threshold below which adverse effects do not occur also applies to these recommended limits.

Additions and Changes to the List of Occupational Exposure Limits

20. The Health and Safety Commission recognizes the need to review exposure limits in the light of new medical and scientific evidence and improvements in engineering control technology. Changes to the list of exposure limits in this Guidance Note will be published by HSE in the Toxic Substances Bulletin and incorporated in the next edition of this Guidance Note.

Long-term and Short-term Exposure Limits

21. Substances hazardous to health may cause adverse effects, e.g. irritation of the skin, eyes or lungs, narcosis or even death after short-term exposure, or via long-term exposure through accumulation of substances in the body or through the gradual development of increased risk of disease with each contact. It is important to control exposure so as to avoid both short-term and long-term effects. Two types of exposure limit are therefore listed. The long-term exposure limit is concerned with the total intake over long periods and is therefore appropriate for protecting against the effects of long-term exposure or reducing the risks to an insignificant level. The short-term exposure limit is aimed primarily at avoiding acute effects, or at least reducing the risk of their occurrence.

22. Both the long-term and short-term exposure limits are expressed as time weighted average (TWA) concentrations which are simply airborne concentrations averaged over a specified period of time. The period for the long-term limit is normally eight hours; when a different period is used this is stated. Some of the short-term exposure limits were formerly expressed as ceiling values, defined as concentrations which should not be exceeded even instantaneously. This cannot be achieved in practice since all samples need to be taken over a finite period of time. A period of ten minutes is considered to be the shortest practicable time over which most personal samples can be taken at the levels of the exposure limits due to the limitations of available sampling and analytical techniques. The short-term exposure limits are therefore normally expressed as 10 minute TWAs. This provides a more accurate indication of exposure because sampling times of less than 10 minutes may fail to detect peaks of shorter duration. In some instances, sampling times of shorter duration may be more appropriate and in such cases this will be stated in the lists.

23. Concentrations of gases and vapours are usually expressed as parts per million (ppm), a measure of concentration by volume, as well as in milligrams per cubic metre of air (mg m^{-3}), a measure of concentration by mass. In converting from ppm to mg m^{-3} a temperature of 25 °C and an atmospheric pressure of one bar were used. Concentrations of airborne particles (fume, dust, etc) are usually expressed in mg m^{-3}, with the exception of asbestos, which is expressed as fibres per millilitre of air (fibres ml^{-1}).

24. This Guidance Note deals primarily with exposure limits for airborne substances. However, when assessing the risk to health for certain substances, e.g. lead, it may be appropriate to supplement the measurements of airborne concentrations with measurements obtained from the analysis of biological

specimens, e.g. levels of the substances or their metabolites in body fluids or in exhaled air obtained from individual workers. Such measurements are known as biological monitoring and indicate an individual worker's 'uptake' or 'response' following exposure. Further information is given in Guidance Note MS 18[2].

Application of Exposure Limits

25. The exposure limits relate to personal exposure (paragraph 39 *et seq.*) with the exception of cotton and vinyl chloride and should be used by employers as guidance for the control of exposure to airborne contamination. They will be taken into account by inspectors when assessing compliance with relevant legal requirements. They should not be used as an index of relative hazard or toxicity. They are not sharp dividing lines between 'safe' and 'dangerous' concentrations nor can they readily be extrapolated to give indications associated with long-term non-occupational exposure, e.g. levels of contamination in the neighbourhood close to an industrial plant.

26. Certain of the exposure limits in this Guidance Note, e.g. those for respirable dusts, carbon dioxide, oxides of nitrogen and carbon monoxide, require special consideration in their application to work in mines and quarries, which are subject to detailed control and practices relevant to those workplaces.

Exposure to all substances, including those listed, should be kept as low as is reasonably practicable at all times. In addition, for listed substances, the exposure limits specified should not normally be exceeded. To help in maintaining operational control it may be appropriate to select action levels, i.e. arbitrary levels at which remedial action is necessary in order to ensure that exposure will remain within the relevant limits.

Mixtures

28. The exposure limits are applicable to airborne concentrations of single substances. Exposure to additional substances, either simultaneously or sequentially, could give rise to greater hazards to health. There is no universally applicable method for the derivation of exposure limits for mixtures from those of individual substances listed in this document. A wide range of formulae of varying degrees of complexity have been devised in recent years for dealing with mixtures; all have limitations and none cope with the problem of synergism (the working together of two or more substances to produce an effect greater than the sum of their individual effects). The suitability of any of these formulae for a particular mixture should be assessed by toxicologists, occupational hygienists and physicians from a specific toxicological consideration of all the substances involved.

Pesticides

29. A number of pesticides are listed either under the trade name of a proprietary formulation or under the common chemical name of the active component. In every case the exposure limit given is for the active component.

Percutaneous Absorption

30. In general, for most substances the main route of entry into the body is by inhalation and the exposure limits given in this Guidance Note are designed to protect the worker agaisnt this risk. Certain substances, marked in the list with an 'Sk' notation, such as phenol, aniline and certain pesticides, have the ability to

penetrate the intact skin and thus become absorbed into the body. Percutaneous absorption (absorption through the skin) can result from local contamination, for example from a splash on the skin or clothing, or in certain cases from exposure to high atmospheric concentrations of vapour. Serious effects can result with little or no warning and it is necessary to take special precautions to prevent skin contact when handling these substances.

Allergenic Sensitizers

31. Other substances may cause allergenic sensitization and give rise to a reaction such as skin rash or an asthmatic condition.[3] Following the induction of a sensitized state, an affected individual may subsequently react to exposure to minute levels of that substance well below the concentrations set out in this list.

Other Factors

32. Any factors which impose additional stress on the body, e.g. long hours of work, exposure to ultraviolet radiation, high temperatures and humidity, may increase the toxic response to a substance. In these circumstances, care must be exercised in the application of the exposure limits listed, as exposure may have to be adjusted to take the effects of these factors into consideration.

Unlisted Substances

33. The absence of a substance from this list does not indicate that it is safe. The policy of HSC is that exposure to any substance, whether or not it is known on present information to be hazardous, should be kept as low as is reasonably practicable. Some substances previously thought to be comparatively safe have subsequently been discovered to pose serious long-term health risks. All substances should, therefore, be handled with care whatever their nature, partly in case future experience shows them to present a hazard which could have been prevented or limited by the application of sensible control measures and partly because sufficient may not be known about their effects in the presence of other substances. Further guidance may be sought from HSE's area offices if necessary.

Monitoring Exposure

34. Where the atmosphere of a workplace is likely to be contaminated, sampling and analysis of the atmosphere may need to be carried out on a periodic basis with a frequency determined by conditions.

35. There are specific legal requirements for the regular measurements of airborne contamination in the Chromium Plating Regulations 1931 (SR and O No 455 as amended by SI 1973 No 9) and in the Control of Lead at Work Regulations 1980 (SI 1980 No 1248).

36. Details of routine sampling strategies for individual substances are outside the scope of this Guidance Note. However, the guidelines below are generally applicable and should prove useful in developing a suitable air sampling strategy to suit most substances and particular circumstances.

37. The development of a routine strategy for monitoring any substance usually involves three steps; (a) a preliminary identification and assessment of the substances liable to be present and an assessment of the hazards which may arise from them; (b) a preliminary survey aimed at identifying the persons exposed to airborne substances and determining their exposure; and (c) using the results of

the preliminary survey to decide on the need for a routine monitoring programme, and if necessary, on its design.

Preliminary Identification and Assessment

38. Work activities should be examined in order to identify the hazardous substances liable to be present and the nature of the hazards which may arise from their presence. On the results of this preliminary identification and assessment the need for a preliminary survey involving atmospheric sampling can be evaluated.

Preliminary Survey

39. All persons exposed to chemical substances in potentially hazardous amounts need to be identified individually. It is important to consider not only those, such as process operators, who may be routinely exposed but also those liable to be intermittently exposed, e.g. maintenance workers, cleaners, crane drivers etc. This exercise requires a detailed knowledge not only of the processes involved and the nature and composition of the substances used, but also the individual tasks of employees.

40. Once the persons likely to be at risk have been identified their exposure should be measured. As the majority of exposure limits relate to personal exposure, personal air sampling techniques should be used initially, with the exceptions given in paragraph 25.

41. In premises where a number of persons are engaged in the same activity, sampling may sometimes be carried out more effectively on a group basis. The persons exposed to substances may be divided into groups engaged in identical or similar work in the same work area. Personal sampling can then be carried out on one or more representative individuals from each group. There may be a variation between the work of each shift, e.g. permanent day and night shifts, in which case each shift should be considered as a separate group.

42. Whether the sampling is being carried out on an individual or on a group basis, the periods over which the samples are taken should be sufficient to give results representative of normal working exposure, including periods of peak and low exposure, so as to enable 8-hour time-weighted average concentrations to be estimated. It is anticipated that in most cases this will entail sampling throughout a normal working day or shift. If sampling shows variation in the day to day working pattern, it will be necessary to sample on several days to cover the normally expected variations. It is important to take account of operations carried out at the beginning and end of the work periods so that operations which may significantly influence the overall exposure level, e.g. weighing-out and machine cleaning, can be included. The results should be reported as 8-hour time-weighted averages (*see* Appendix 1a). Similarly, it is also important to take account of operations where peak concentrations are likely to occur when assessing short-term exposure.

43. Valuable additional information about variation of exposure within shifts may be obtained by splitting the sampling period into separate shorter duration sampling periods around natural breaks in the shift, e.g. meal breaks. The results of these shorter duration samples should be suitably combined on a time-weighted average basis to estimate the longer term 8-hour exposures (*see* Appendix 1b).

44. Static sampling can be carried out in the work areas to supplement personal sampling. This will provide information on the relationship between personal

samples and the concentration of airborne contaminants at fixed points and will enable the role of static sampling in future air monitoring programmes to be determined. However, if static sampling is to be used instead of personal sampling, employers should be able to demonstrate that personal exposures are not higher than the concentrations at the static sampling locations in the work area in question or that the ratio of static to personal sampling results is fairly constant so that a reliable estimate of personal exposure can be made.

Routine Monitoring

45. The preliminary survey will enable the details of the routine monitoring programme to be established, such as deciding the number and location of sampling points (personal and static), the balance required between personal and static sampling where both methods are used and the frequency at which subsequent routine monitoring should be carried out. Personal sampling on a routine basis should be carried out as for the preliminary survey. However, where the preliminary survey or other results show that there is a consistently satisfactory pattern of exposure to airborne contaminants, it may be appropriate to reduce the frequency at which sampling is carried out and/or the length of sampling time during routine sampling, so long as it covers a representative period.

46. Sufficient samples should be taken during routine monitoring to enable any major changes in exposure levels to be identified. Any individual results above the exposure should be carefully investigated and steps taken to reduce exposure to as low as is reasonably practicable and within the exposure limits. For groups, the results should be compared with the results of the preliminary survey and any other results from the same group. Abnormal results should be investigated further and appropriate corrective action taken.

47. Where exposure is intermittent, it is recommended that the sampling periods should be designed to coincide with specific operations so that satisfactory time-weighted averages for both the long-term and short-term exposures of work people can be calculated (*see* Appendix 1c).

48. The routine air monitoring programme should be reviewed in the light of experience, if any new processes are introduced, or if other changes occur that might affect the pattern and degree of exposure. Results from air monitoring exercises should be recorded and retained as they provide information on the effectiveness of control procedures and may be useful for epidemiological studies.

Sampling and Analytical Techniques

49. The sampling and analytical techniques used for a monitoring programme are usually influenced by its objectives. Establishing personal exposure, determining the nature and concentrations of contaminants in the work environment, investigating patterns of exposure or checking the effectiveness of control measures in reducing personal exposure may require different techniques.

50. Advice on methods of sampling and analysis of certain substances is given in *Methods for the Determination of Hazardous Substances*. These publications are listed on p. 145. Advice on the sampling of asbestos, cotton dust, PVC dust, talc and lead is given in Guidance Notes.

51. Further advice may be obtained from HSE inspectors or from occupational hygienists, toxicologists or occupational physicians.

Further Advice

52. Scientific information, exposure data and literature references pertinent to the substances listed may be found in the toxicology reviews published by HSE[4] and the documentation accompanying other national lists.[5,6]

53. A full range of HSE literature may be found in the *Publications Catalogue*, available from Her Majesty's Stationery Office or through booksellers.

List of Occupational Exposure Limits

Annotations   Sk   Can be absorbed through the skin

ISO   International Organisation for Standardisation

INN   International Non-proprietary Name

Part 1: Control limits (paragraph 15)

Substance	Formula	Long-term exposure limit (8-hour TWA value)		Short-term exposure limit (10 minutes TWA value)		Notes
		ppm	mg m^{-3}	ppm	mg m^{-3}	
Acrylonitrile	$CH_2=CHCN$	2	4	—	—	Sk
Asbestos	*see Guidance Note EH 10[9]*					
Carbon disulphide	CS_2	10	30	—	—	Sk
Coal dust, in mines	*see Appendix 4*					
Ethylene oxide	CH_2CH_2O	5	10	—	—	
Isocyanates, all (as-NCO)	*See Appendix 2*	—	0·02	—	0·07	
Lead and compounds		100	420	250	1050	from 1.4.84
Styrene	$C_6H_5CH=CH_2$					
Trichloroethylene	$CCl_2=CHCl$	100	535	150	802	Sk
Vinyl chloride (Chloroethylene)	*See Appendix 3*					

Part 2: Recommended limits (paragraph 18)

Substance	Formula	Long-term exposure limit (8-hour TWA value)		Short-term exposure limit (10-minute TWA value)		Notes
		ppm	$mg\,m^{-3}$	ppm	$mg\,m^{-3}$	
Acetaldehyde	CH_3CHO	100	180	150	270	
Acetic acid	CH_3COOH	10	25	15	37	
Acetic anhydride	$(CH_3CO)_2O$	5	20	5	20	
Acetone	CH_3COCH_3	1000	2400	1250	3000	
Acetonitrile	CH_3CN	40	70	60	105	
o-Acetylsalicylic acid	$CH_3COOC_6H_4COOH$	—	5	—	—	
Acrolein	see Acrylaldehyde					
Acrylaldehyde	$CH_2{=}CHCHO$	0·1	0·25	0·3	0·8	
Acrylamide	$CH_2{=}CHCONH_2$	—	0·3	—	0·6	Sk
Acrylonitrile	see Part 1 for control limit					
Aldrin (ISO)	$C_{12}H_8Cl_6$	—	0·25	—	0·75	Sk
Allyl alcohol	$CH_2{=}CHCH_2OH$	2	5	4	10	Sk
Allyl chloride	see 3-Chloropropene					
Allyl 2,3-epoxypropyl ether	$CH_2{=}CHCH_2OCH_2\underset{\text{O}}{CHCH_2}$	5	22	10	44	Sk
Allyl glycidyl ether (AGE)	see Allyl 2,3-epoxypropyl ether					
Aluminium alkyl compounds		2	—	—	—	
Aluminium metal and oxide	$Al;Al_2O_3$	—	10	—	20	
Aluminium salts, soluble		—	2	—	—	
2-Aminoethanol	$NH_2CH_2CH_2OH$	3	8	6	15	
2-Aminopyridine	see 2-Pyridylamine					
Ammonia	NH_3	25	18	35	27	
Ammonium chloride, fume	NH_4Cl	—	10	—	20	
Ammonium sulphamidate	$NH_2SO_3NH_4$	—	10	—	20	
n-Amyl acetate	see Pentyl acetate					
sec-Amyl acetate	see 1-Methylbutyl acetate					
Aniline	$C_6H_5NH_2$	2	10	5	20	Sk
Anisidines, o and p-isomers	$NH_2C_6H_4OCH_3$	0·1	0·5	—	—	Sk
Antimony & compounds (as Sb)	Sb	—	0·5	—	—	

Substance	Formula					
Arsenic & compounds, except arsine and lead arsenate, (as As)	As	—	0·2	—	—	
Arsine	AsH_3	0·05	0·2	—	—	
Asbestos, all forms	*see Part 1 for control limits*					
Asphalt, petroleum fumes		—	5	—	10	
Aspirin	*see o-Acetylsalicylic acid*					
Atrazine (ISO)	$C_8H_{14}ClN_5$	—	10	—	—	
Azinphos-methyl (ISO)	$(CH_3O)_2PSSCH_2(C_7H_4N_3O)$	—	0·2	—	0·6	Sk
Aziridine	$\overline{CH_2CH_2NH}$	0·5	1	—	—	Sk
γ-BHC (ISO)	$C_6H_6Cl_6$	—	0·5	—	1·5	Sk
Barium compounds, soluble (as Ba)	Ba	—	0·5	—	—	
Barium sulphate, respirable dust (see Appendix 4)	$BaSO_4$	—	4	—	—	
Benomyl (ISO)	$C_{14}H_{18}N_4O_3$	—	10	—	15	
Benzene	C_6H_6	10	30	—	—	
Benzene-1,2,4-tricarboxylic acid 1,2-anhydride	$C_9H_4O_5$	—	0·04	—	—	
p-Benzoquinone	$C_6H_4O_2$	0·1	0·4	0·3	1·2	
Benzoyl peroxide	*see Dibenzoyl peroxide*					
Benzyl chloride	*see α-Chlorotoluene*					
Beryllium	Be	—	0·002	—	—	
Biphenyl	$(C_6H_5)_2$	0·2	1·5	0·6	4	
Bis(chloromethyl) ether	$ClCH_2OCH_2Cl$	0·001	—	—	—	
2,2-Bis(p-chlorophenyl)-1,1,1-trichloroethane	*see 1,1,1-Trichlorobis(chlorophenyl)ethane*					
Bis(2,3-epoxypropyl) ether	$(CH_2CHCH_2)_2O$	0·5	3	0·5	3	
Bis(2-ethylhexyl) phthalate	$C_6H_4[COOCH_2CH(C_2H_5)C_4H_9]_2$	—	5	—	10	
2,2-Bis(p-methoxyphenyl)-1,1,1-trichloroethane	*see Methoxychlor (ISO)*					
Bismuth telluride	*see Dibismuth trielluride*					
Bismuth telluride, selenium-doped	*see Dibismuth trielluride, selenium-doped*					
Borates, (tetra) sodium salts,	*see Disodium tetraborate*					
Bornan-2-one	$C_{10}H_{16}O$	2	12	3	18	
Boron oxide	*see Diboron trioxide*					
Boron tribromide	BBr_3	1	10	3	30	
Boron trifluoride	BF_3	1	3	1	3	

Substance	Formula	Long-term exposure limit (8-hour TWA value)		Short-term exposure limit (10-minute TWA value)		Notes
		ppm	mg m^{-3}	ppm	mg m^{-3}	
Bromacil (ISO)	$C_9H_{13}BrN_2O_2$	1	10	2	20	
Bromine	Br_2	0·1	0·7	0·3	2	
Bromine pentafluoride	BrF_5	0·1	0·7	0·3	2	
Bromochloromethane	CH_2BrCl	200	1050	250	1300	
Bromoethane	C_2H_5Br	200	890	250	1110	
Bromoethylene	CH_2CHBr	5	20	—	—	Sk
Bromoform	$CHBr_3$	0·5	5	—	—	Sk
Bromomethane	CH_3Br	15	60	—	—	
Bromotrifluoromethane	CF_3Br	1000	6100	1200	7300	
Buta-1,3-diene	$CH_2{=}CHCH{=}CH_2$	1000	2200	1250	2750	Sk
Butane	C_4H_{10}	600	1430	750	1780	
Butan-1-ol	$CH_3CH_2CH_2CH_2OH$	50	150	50	150	Sk
Butan-2-ol	$CH_3CH_2CHOHCH_3$	150	450	—	—	
Butan-2-one	$CH_3COC_2H_5$	200	590	300	885	
trans-But-2-enal	$CH_3CH{=}CHCHO$	2	6	6	18	
2-Butoxyethanol	$C_4H_9OCH_2CH_2OH$	50	240	150	720	Sk
Butyl acetate	$CH_3COO(CH_2)_3CH_3$	150	710	200	950	
sec-Butyl acetate	$CH_3COOCH(CH_3)CH_2CH_3$	200	950	250	1190	
tert-Butyl acetate	$CH_3COOC(CH_3)_3$	200	950	250	1190	
Butyl acrylate	$C_7H_{12}O_2$	10	55	—	—	
n-Butyl alcohol	see Butan-1-ol					
sec-Butyl alcohol	see Butan-2-ol					
tert-Butyl alcohol	see 2-Methylpropan-2-ol					
Butylamine	$CH_3CH_2CH_2CH_2NH_2$	5	15	5	15	Sk
Butyl 2,3-epoxypropyl ether	$C_4H_9OCH_2CHCH_2$ (epoxide)	50	270	—	—	
n-Butylglycidyl ether (BGE)	see Butyl 2,3-epoxypropyl ether					
Butyl lactate	$C_7H_{14}O_3$	5	25	—	—	

Substance	Formula					
Cadmium, dust & salts (as Cd)	Cd	—	0·05	—	0·2	
Cadmium oxide, fume (as Cd)	CdO	—	0·05	—	0·05	
Caesium hydroxide	$CsOH$	—	2	—	—	
Calcium cyanamide	$CaNC{\equiv}N$	—	0·5	—	1	
Calcium hydroxide	$Ca(OH)_2$	—	5	—	—	
Calcium oxide	CaO	—	2	—	—	
Camphor, synthetic	*see Bornan-2-one*					
ε-Caprolactam	$CH_2CH_2CH_2NH$ / CH_2CH_2CO					
dust		—	1	—	3	
vapour		5	20	10	40	
Captafol (ISO)	$C_{10}H_9Cl_4NO_2S$	—	0·1	—	—	Sk
Captan (ISO)	$C_9H_8Cl_3NO_2S$	—	5	—	15	
Carbaryl (ISO)	$C_{10}H_7OCONHCH_3$	—	5	—	10	
Carbofuran (ISO)	$C_{12}H_{15}NO_3$	—	0·1	—	—	
Carbon black	C	—	3·5	—	7	
Carbon dioxide	CO_2	5000	9000	15000	27000	
Carbon disulphide	*see Part 1 for control limit*					
Carbon monoxide	CO	50	55	400	440	
Carbon tetrabromide	CBr_4	0·1	1·4	0·3	4	
Carbon tetrachloride	CCl_4	10	65	20	130	Sk
Carbonyl chloride	*see Phosgene*					
Catechol	*see Pyrocatechol*					
Cellulose		—	10	—	20	
Chlordane (ISO)	$C_{10}H_6Cl_8$	—	0·5	—	2	Sk
Chlorinated biphenyls (42% chlorine)	$C_{12}H_7Cl_3$ (approx)	—	1	—	2	Sk
Chlorinated biphenyls (54% chlorine)	$C_6H_2Cl_3C_6H_3Cl_2$	—	0·5	—	1	Sk
Chlorine	Cl_2	1	3	3	9	
Chlorine dioxide	ClO_2	0·1	0·3	0·3	0·9	
Chlorine trifluoride	ClF_3	0·1	0·4	0·1	0·4	
Chloroacetaldehyde	$ClCH_2CHO$	1	3	1	3	
2-Chloroacetophenone	$C_6H_5COCH_2Cl$	0·05	0·3	—	—	
Chloroacetyl chloride	$ClCH_2OCl$	0·05	0·2	—	—	
Chlorobenzene	C_6H_5Cl	75	350	—	—	
Chlorobromomethane	*see Bromochloromethane*					
2-Chlorobuta-1,3-diene	$CH_2{=}CClCH{=}CH_2$	10	36	—	—	Sk
Chlorodifluoromethane	$CHClF_2$	1000	3500	1250	4375	
1-Chloro-2,3-epoxy-propane	OCH_2CHCH_2Cl	2	8	5	20	Sk
Chloroethane	C_2H_5Cl	1000	2600	1250	3250	

Substance	Formula	Long-term exposure limit (8-hour TWA value)		Short-term exposure limit (10-minute TWA value)		Notes
		ppm	mg m^{-3}	ppm	mg m^{-3}	
2-Chloroethanol	ClCH$_2$CH$_2$OH	1	3	1	3	Sk
Chloroethylene	*see Part 1 for control limit*					
Chloroform	CHCl$_3$	10	50	50	225	
Chloromethane	CH$_3$Cl	100	210	125	260	
1-Chloro-4-nitrobenzene	ClC$_6$H$_4$NO$_2$	—	1	—	2	Sk
Chloropicrin	*see Trichloronitromethane*					
β-Chloroprene	*see 2-Chlorobuta-1,3-diene*					
3-Chloropropene	CH$_2$=CHCH$_2$Cl	1	3	2	6	
α-Chlorotoluene	C$_6$H$_5$CH$_2$Cl	1	5	—	—	
2-Chloro-6-(trichloro-methyl) pyridine	C$_6$H$_3$Cl$_4$N	—	10	—	20	
Chloropyrifos (ISO)	C$_9$H$_{11}$Cl$_3$NO$_3$PS	—	0.2	—	0.6	Sk
Chromium	Cr	—	0.5	—	—	
Chromium (II) compounds (as Cr)	Cr	—	0.5	—	—	
Chromium (III) compounds (as Cr)	Cr	—	0.5	—	—	
Chromium (VI) compounds (as Cr)	Cr	—	0.05	—	—	
Coal dust, containing <5% quartz, respirable dust (see Appendix 4)						
Coal dust, containing >5% quartz	*see Appendix 4*	—	2	—	—	
Coal dust, in mines	*see Part 1 for control limit*					
Coal tar pitch volatiles (as benzene solubles)		—	0.2	—	—	
Cobalt & compounds (as Co)	Co	—	0.1	—	—	
Copper, fume	Cu	—	0.2	—	—	
dusts and mists		—	1	—	2	
Cotton dust	*see Appendix 4*					
Cresols, all isomers	CH$_3$C$_6$H$_4$OH	5	22	—	—	Sk
Cristobalite, total dust	SiO$_2$	—	0.15	—	—	
respirable dust (see Appendix 4)		—	0.05	—	—	

Crotonaldehyde	*see trans-But-2-enal*					
Cryofluorane (INN)	$CClF_2CClF_2$	1000	7000	1250	8750	Sk
Cumene	$C_6H_5CH(CH_3)_2$	50	245	75	365	
Cyanamide	$H_2NC{\equiv}N$	—	2	—	—	
Cyanides, except hydrogen cyanide, cyanogen & cyanogen chloride, (as -CN)		—	5	—	—	Sk
Cyanogen	*see Oxalonitrile*					
Cyanogen chloride	$ClCN$	0·3	0·6	0·3	0·6	
Cyclohexane	C_6H_{12}	300	1050	375	1300	
Cyclohexanol	$C_6H_{11}OH$	50	200	—	—	
Cyclohexanone	$C_6H_{10}O$	50	200	—	—	
Cyclohexene	C_6H_{10}	300	1015	—	—	
Cyclonite (RDX)	*see 1,3,5-Trinitro-1,3,5-triazinane*					
Cyhexatin (ISO)	$(C_6H_{11})_3SnOH$	—	5	—	10	
2,4-D (ISO)	$C_6H_3Cl_2OCH_2COOH$	—	10	—	20	
DDT	*see 1,1,1-Trichlorobis(chlorophenyl) ethane*					
DDVP	*see Dichlorvos (ISO)*					
2,4-DES	*see Sodium 2-(2,4-dichlorophenoxy) ethyl sulphate*					
DMDT	*see Methoxychlor (ISO)*					
Derris, commercial	*see Rotenone*					
Diacetone alcohol	*see 4-Hydroxy-4-methylpentan-2-one*					
2,2'-Diaminodiethylamine	*see 2,2'-Iminodi(ethylamine)*					
4,4'-Diaminodiphenyl-methane (DADPM)	*see 4,4'-Methylenedianiline*					
1,2-Diaminoethane	*see Ethylenediamine*					
Diatomaceous earth, natural, respirable dust (see Appendix 4)						
Diazinon (ISO)	$C_{12}H_{21}N_2O_3PS$	—	1·5	—	—	Sk
Diazomethane	$CH_2{=}N_2$	0·2	0·1	—	0·3	
Dibenzoyl peroxide	$(C_6H_5CO)_2O_2$	—	0·4	—	—	
Dibismuth tritelluride	Bi_2Te_3	—	5	—	20	
Dibismuth tritelluride, selenium doped	Bi_2Te_3	—	10	—	10	
Diborane	B_2H_6	0·1	5	—	—	
Diboron trioxide	B_2O_3	—	0·1	—	20	
Dibrom	*see Naled (ISO)*					

Substance	Formula	Long-term exposure limit (8-hour TWA value)		Short-term exposure limit (10-minute TWA value)		Notes
		ppm	$mg\ m^{-3}$	ppm	$mg\ m^{-3}$	
1,2-Dibromo-2,2-dichloroethyl dimethyl phosphate	see Naled (ISO)					
Dibromodifluoromethane	CBr_2F_2	100	860	150	1290	
Dibutyl hydrogen phosphate	$(n\text{-}C_4H_9O)_2(OH)PO$	1	5	2	10	
Di-n-butyl phosphate	see Dibutyl hydrogen phosphate					
Dibutyl phthalate	$C_6H_4(CO_2C_4H_9)_2$	—	5	—	10	
6,6'-Di-tert-butyl-4,4'-thiodi-m-cresol	$C_{22}H_{30}O_2S$	—	10	—	20	
Dichloroacetylene	$ClC{\equiv}CCl$	0·1	0·4	0·1	0·4	
1,2-Dichlorobenzene	$C_6H_4Cl_2$	50	300	50	300	
1,4-Dichlorobenzene	$C_6H_4Cl_2$	75	450	110	675	
Dichlorodifluoromethane	CCl_2F_2	1000	4950	1250	6200	
1,3-Dichloro-5,5-dimethyl-hydantoin	$C_5H_6Cl_2N_2O_2$	—	0·2	—	0·4	
Dichlorodiphenyl-trichloroethane	see 1,1,1-Trichlorobis(chlorophenyl) ethane					
1,1-Dichloroethane	CH_3CHCl_2	200	810	250	1010	
1,2-Dichloroethane	CH_2ClCH_2Cl	10	40	15	60	
1,1-Dichloroethylene	$CH_2{=}CCl_2$	10	40	20	80	
1,2-Dichloroethylene,cis:trans isomers 60:40	$ClCH{=}CHCl$	200	790	250	1000	
Dichlorofluoromethane	$CHCl_2F$	10	40	—	—	
Dichloromethane	CH_2Cl_2	200	700	250	870	
2,2'-Dichloro-4,4'-methylene-dianiline	$CH_2(C_6H_3ClNH_2)_2$	—	0·05	—	—	Sk
2,4-Dichlorophenoxyacetic acid	see 2,4-D (ISO)					
1,3-Dichloropropene,cis and trans isomers	$CHCl{=}CHCH_2Cl$	1	5	10	50	Sk
1,2-Dichlorotetra-fluoroethane	see Cryofluorane (INN)					
Dichlorvos (ISO)	$(CH_3O)_2POOCH{=}CCl_2$	0·1	1	0·3	3	Sk
Dicyclopentadienyliron	see Ferrocene					
Dieldrin (ISO)	$C_{12}H_8Cl_6O$	—	0·25	—	0·75	Sk
Diethylamine	$(C_2H_5)_2NH$	25	75	—	—	
2-Diethylaminoethanol	$(C_2H_5)_2NCH_2CH_2OH$	10	50	—	—	Sk
Diethylene triamine	see 2,2'-1minodi(ethylamine)					

		400	1200	500	1500	Sk
Diethyl ether	$C_2H_5OC_2H_5$	400	1200	500	1500	
Di-2-ethylhexyl phthalate	see Bis(2-ethylhexyl) phthalate					
Diethyl ketone	see Pentan-3-one					
Diethyl phthalate	$C_6H_4(COOC_2H_5)_2$	—	5	—	10	
Difluorochloromethane	see Chlorodifluoromethane					
Difluorodibromomethane	see Dibromodifluoromethane					
Difluorodichloromethane	see Dichlorodifluoromethane					
Diglycidyl ether (DGE)	see Bis(2,3-epoxypropyl) ether					
o-Dihydroxybenzene	see Pyrocatechol					
m-Dihydroxybenzene	see Resorcinol					
p-Dihydroxybenzene	see Hydroquinone					
1,2-Dihydroxyethane	see Ethane-1,2-diol					
Di-isobutyl ketone	see 2,6-Dimethylheptan-4-one					
Di-isopropylamine	$(CH_3)_2CHNHCH(CH_3)_2$	5	20	—	—	Sk
Di-isopropyl ether	$(CH_3)_2CHOCH(CH_3)_2$	250	1050	310	1320	
Dimethoxymethane	$CH_2(OCH_3)_2$	1000	3100	1250	3875	
N,N-Dimethylacetamide	$CH_3CON(CH_3)_2$	10	35	15	50	Sk
Dimethylamine	$(CH_3)_2NH$	10	18			
N,N-Dimethylaniline	$C_6H_5N(CH_3)_2$	5	25	10	50	Sk
Dimethylformamide	$HCON(CH_3)_2$	10	30	20	60	Sk
2,6-Dimethylheptan-4-one	$[(CH_3)_2CHCH_2]_2CO$	25	150			
Dimethyl phthalate	$C_6H_4(COOCH_3)_2$	—	5	—	10	Sk
Dimethyl sulphate	$(CH_3)_2SO_4$	0·1	0·5	0·1	0·5	Sk
Dinitrobenzene, all isomers	$C_6H_4(NO_2)_2$	0·15	1	0·5	3	
Dinitro-o-cresol	see 2-Methyl-4,6-dinitrophenol					
2,4-Dinitrotoluene	$CH_3C_6H_3(NO_2)_2$	—	1·5	—	5	Sk
Di-sec-octyl phthalate	see Bis(2-ethylhexyl) phthalate					
1,4-Dioxane, tech. grade	$\overline{OCH_2CH_2OCH_2CH_2}$	50	180	—	—	Sk
Dioxathion (ISO)	$C_{12}H_{26}O_6P_2S_2$	—	0·2	—	—	Sk
Diphenyl	see Biphenyl					
Diphenylamine	$(C_6H_5)_2NH$	—	10	—	20	
Diphosphorus pentasulphide	P_2S_5	—	1	—	3	
Diquat dibromide (ISO)	$C_{12}H_{12}Br_2N_2$	—	0·5	—	1	
Disodium disulphite	$Na_2S_2O_5$	—	5	—	—	

Substance	Formula	Long-term exposure limit (8-hour TWA value)		Short-term exposure limit (10-minute TWA value)		Notes
		ppm	mg m⁻³	ppm	mg m⁻³	
Disodium tetraborate,						
anhydrous	$Na_2B_4O_7$	—	1	—	—	
decahydrate	$Na_2B_4O_7 \cdot 10H_2O$	—	5	—	—	
penntahydrate	$Na_2B_4O_7 \cdot 5H_2O$	—	1	—	—	
Disulfoton (ISO)	$(C_2H_5O)_2PSCH_2CH_2SC_2H_5$	—	0·1	—	0·3	
Disulphur dichloride	S_2Cl_2	1	6	3	18	
Disulphur decafluoride	S_2F_{10}	0·025	0·25	0·075	0·75	
Diuron (ISO)	$C_9H_{10}Cl_2N_2O$	—	10	—	—	
Divanadium pentaoxide (as V),	V_2O_5					
dust		—	0·5	—	1·5	
fume		—	0·05	—	0·05	
Dust, not otherwise specified						
total dust		—	10	—	—	
respirable dust (see Appendix 4)		—	5	—	—	
Endosulfan (ISO)	$C_9H_6Cl_6O_3S$	—	0·1	—	0·3	Sk
Endrin (ISO)	$C_{12}H_8Cl_6O$	—	0·1	—	0·3	Sk
Epichlorohydrin	*see 1-Chloro-2,3-epoxypropane*					
1,2-Epoxy-4-epoxyethyl-cyclohexane	$C_8H_{12}O_2$	10	60	—	—	
1,2-Epoxypropane	CH_3CHCH_2O	100	240	150	360	
2,3-Epoxypropyl isopropyl ether	$C_3H_7\text{-}OCH_2CHCH_2\,O$	50	240	75	360	
Ethane-1,2-diol,						
particulate	CH_2OHCH_2OH	—	10	—	20	
vapour		100	250	125	325	
Ethanethiol	C_2H_5SH	0·5	1	2	3	
Ethanol	C_2H_5OH	1000	1900	—	—	

Substance	Formula / Reference					
Ethanolamine	*see 2-Aminoethanol*					
Ether	*see Diethyl ether*					
2-Ethoxyethanol	$C_2H_5OCH_2CH_2OH$	100	370	150	560	Sk
2-Ethoxyethyl acetate	$C_2H_5OCH_2CH_2OOCCH_3$	100	540	150	810	Sk
Ethyl acetate	$CH_3COOC_2H_5$	400	1400	—	—	
Ethyl acrylate	$CH_2{=}CHCOOC_2H_5$	25	100			
Ethyl alcohol	*see Ethanol*					
Ethylamine	$C_2H_5NH_2$	10	18			
Ethyl amyl ketone	*see 5-Methylheptan-3-one*					
Ethylbenzene	$C_6H_5C_2H_5$	100	435	125	545	
Ethyl bromide	*see Bromoethane*					
Ethyl butyl ketone	*see Heptan-3-one*					
Ethyl chloride	*see Chloroethane*					
Ethylene chlorohydrin	*see 2-Chloroethanol*					
Ethylenediamine	$NH_2CH_2CH_2NH_2$	10	25	—	—	Sk
Ethylene dichloride	*see 1,2-Dichloroethane*					
Ethylene dinitrate	$CH_2NO_3CH_2NO_3$	0·2	2	0·2	2	Sk
Ethylene glycol	*see Ethane-1,2-diol*					
Ethylene glycol dinitrate (EGDN)	*see Ethylene dinitrate*					
Ethylene glycol monobutyl ether	*see 2-Butoxyethanol*					
Ethylene glycol monoethyl ether acetate	*see 2-Ethoxyethyl acetate*					
Ethylene glycol monoethyl ether	*see 2-Ethoxyethanol*					
Ethylene glycol monomethyl ether acetate	*see 2-Methoxyethyl acetate*					
Ethylene glycol monomethyl ether	*see 2-Methoxyethanol*					
Ethylene oxide	*see Part 1 for control limit*					
Ethylenimine	*see Aziridine*					
Ethyl ether	*see Diethyl ether*					
Ethyl formate	$HCOOC_2H_5$	100	300	150	450	
Ethylidene dichloride	*see 1,1-Dichloroethane*					
Ethyl mercaptan	*see Ethanethiol*					
4-Ethylmorpholine	$C_6H_{13}NO$	20	95	—	—	Sk
Ethyl silicate	*see Tetraethyl orthosilicate*					
Fenchlorphos (ISO)	$(CH_3O)_2PSOC_6H_2Cl_3$	—	10	—	—	
Ferbam (ISO)	$[(CH_3)_2NCSS]_3Fe$	—	10	—	20	
Ferrocene	$C_{10}H_{10}Fe$	—	10	—	20	
Fluoride (as F)	F	—	2·5	—	—	
Fluorine	F_2	1	2	2	4	

Substance	Formula	Long-term exposure limit (8-hour TWA value)		Short-term exposure limit (10-minute TWA value)		Notes
		ppm	mg m^{-3}	ppm	mg m^{-3}	
Fluorodichloromethane	*see Dichlorofluoromethane*					
Fluorotrichloromethane	*see Trichlorofluoromethane*					
Formaldehyde	HCHO	2	3	2	3	Sk
Formamide	HCONH$_2$	20	30	30	45	Sk
Formic acid	HCOOH	5	9	—	—	
2-Furaldehyde (Furfural)	C$_5$H$_4$O$_2$	5	20	15	60	
Furfuryl alcohol	OCH=CHCH=CCH$_2$OH	5	20	10	40	
Germane	GeH$_4$	0·2	0·6	0·6	1·8	
Germanium tetrahydride	*see Germane*					
Glutaraldehyde	OCH(CH$_2$)$_3$CHO	0·2	0·7	0·2	0·7	Sk
Glycerol, mist	CH$_2$OHCHOHCH$_2$OH	—	10	—	20	
Glycerol trinitrate	CH$_2$NO$_3$CHNO$_3$CH$_2$NO$_3$	0·2	2	0·2	2	
Glycol monoethyl ether	*see 2-Ethoxyethanol*					
Graphite, containing <1% quartz total dust	C	—	10	—	—	
respirable dust (see Appendix 4)		—	5	—	—	
Graphite, containing >1% quartz	*see Appendix 4*					
Guthion	*see Azinphos-methyl (ISO)*					
γ-HCH (ISO)	*see γ-BHC (ISO)*					
Hafnium	HF	—	0·5	—	1·5	
Heptachlor (ISO)	C$_{10}$H$_5$Cl$_7$	—	0·5	—	2	Sk
n-Heptane	C$_7$H$_{16}$	400	1600	500	2000	
Heptan-3-one	CH$_3$CH$_2$CO(CH$_2$)$_3$CH$_3$	50	230	75	345	
γ-Hexachlorocyclohexane	*see γ-BHC (ISO)*					
Hexachloroethane	CCl$_3$CCl$_3$	1	10	3	30	Sk
n-Hexane	C$_6$H$_{14}$	100	360	125	450	
Hexan-2-one	CH$_3$(CH$_2$)$_3$COCH$_3$	25	100	40	165	Sk
Hexone	*see 4-Methylpentan-2-one*					

Substance	Formula					
Hydrazine	NH_2NH_2	0·1	0·1	—	—	Sk
Hydrogen bromide	HBr	3	10	—	—	
Hydrogen chloride	HCl	5	7	5	7	
Hydrogen cyanide	HCN	10	10	10	10	Sk
Hydrogen fluoride (as F)	HF	3	2·5	6	5	
Hydrogen peroxide	H_2O_2	1	1·5	2	3	
Hydrogen selenide (as Se)	H_2Se	0·05	0·2	—	—	
Hydrogen sulphide	H_2S	10	14	15	21	
Hydroquinone	$C_6H_4(OH)_2$	—	2	—	4	
4-Hydroxy-4-methyl-pentan-2-one	$CH_3COCH_2C(CH_3)_2OH$	50	240	75	360	
2-Hydroxypropyl acrylate	$CH_2CHCOOCH_2CHOHCH_3$	0·5	3	—	—	Sk
2,2'-Iminodi(ethylamine)	$(NH_2CH_2CH_2)_2NH$	1	4	—	—	Sk
Indene	C_9H_8	10	45	15	70	
Indium & compounds (as In)	In	—	0·1	—	0·3	
Iodine	I_2	0·1	1	0·1	1	
Iodoform	CHI_3	0·6	10	1	20	
Iodomethane	CH_3I	5	28	10	56	Sk
Iron oxide, fume (as Fe)	Fe_2O_3	—	5	—	10	
Iron pentacarbonyl	see Pentacarbonyl iron					
Iron salts (as Fe)	Fe	—	1	—	2	
Isoamyl acetate	see Isopentyl acetate					
Isoamyl alcohol	see 3-Methylbutan-1-ol					
Isoamyl methyl ketone	see 5-Methylhexan-2-one					
Isocyanates, all	see Part 1 for control limit					
Isobutyl acetate	$CH_3COOCH_2CH(CH_3)_2$	150	700	187	875	
Isobutyl alcohol	see 2-Methylpropan-1-ol					
Isobutyl methyl ketone	see 4-Methylpentan-2-one					
Isopentyl acetate	$CH_3COOCH_2CH_2CH(CH_3)_2$	100	525	125	655	
Isophorone	see 3,5,5-Trimethylcyclohex-2-enone					
Isophorone diisocyanate (IPDI)	see Part 1 for control limit					
Isopropyl acetate	$CH_3COOCH(CH_3)_2$	250	950	310	1185	
Isopropyl alcohol	see Propan-2-ol					
Isopropyl benzene	see Cumene					
Isopropyl ether	see Diisopropyl ether					
Isopropyl glycidyl ether (IGE)	see 2,3-Epoxypropyl isopropyl ether					

Substance	Formula	Long-term exposure limit (8-hour TWA value)		Short-term exposure limit (10-minute TWA value)		Notes
		ppm	mg m^{-3}	ppm	mg m^{-3}	
Ketene	$CH_2{=}CO$	0·5	0·9	1·5	3	
Lead and compounds	*see Part 1 for control limit*					
Lindane	*see γ-BHC (ISO)*					
Liquefied petroleum gas (LPG)	Mixture: C_5H_6; C_3H_8; C_4H_8; C_4H_{10}	1000	1800	1250	2250	
Lithium hydride	LiH	—	0·025	—	—	
MbOCA	*see 2,2'-Dichloro-4,4' methylene-dianiline*					
Magnesium oxide, fume (as Mg)	MgO	—	10	—	—	
Malathion (ISO)	$C_{10}H_{19}O_6PS_2$	—	10	—	—	Sk
Maleic anhydride	$C_4H_2O_3$	0·25	1	—	—	
Manganese, fume (as Mn)	Mn	—	1	—	3	
Manganese and compounds (as Mn)		—	5	—	5	
Manganese cyclopentadienyl tricarbonyl	*see Tricarbonyl(eta-cyclopentadienyl) manganese*					
Manganese tetroxide	*see Trimanganese tetraoxide*					
Mercaptoacetic acid	$C_2H_4O_2S$	1	5	—	—	Sk
Mercury alkyls (as Hg)		—	0·01	—	0·03	Sk
Mercury & compounds, except mercury alkyls, (as Hg)	Hg	—	0·05	—	0·15	
Mesityl oxide	*see 4-Methylpent-3-en-2-one*					
Methanethiol	CH_3SH	0·5	1	—	—	
Methanol	CH_3OH	200	260	250	310	Sk
Methomyl (ISO)	$C_5H_{10}N_2O_2S$	—	2·5	—	—	Sk
Methoxychlor (ISO)	$C_{16}H_{15}Cl_3O_2$	—	10	—	—	
2-Methoxyethanol	$CH_3OCH_2CH_2OH$	25	80	35	120	Sk

2-Methoxyethyl acetate	$CH_3COOCH_2CH_2OCH_3$	25	120	35	170	Sk
1-Methoxypropan-2-ol	$CH_3OCH_2CHOHCH_3$	100	360	150	540	
Methyl acetate	CH_3COOCH_3	200	610	250	760	Sk
Methyl acrylate	$CH_2=CHCOOCH_3$	10	35	—	—	
Methylal	*see Dimethoxymethane*					
Methyl alcohol	*see Methanol*					
Methylamine	CH_3NH_2	10	12	—	—	
Methyl amyl alcohol	*see 4-Methylpentan-2-ol*					
Methyl bromide	*see Bromomethane*					
3-Methylbutan-1-ol	$(CH_3)_2CHCH_2CH_2OH$	100	360	125	450	
1-Methylbutyl acetate	$CH_3COOCH(CH_3)C_3H_7$	125	670	150	800	
Methylbutyl ketone	*see Hexan-2-one*					
Methyl chloride	*see Chloromethane*					
Methyl chloroform	*see 1,1,1-Trichloroethane*					
Methyl 2-cyanoacrylate	$CH_2=C(CN)COOCH_3$	2	8	4	16	
Methylcyclohexanols	$CH_3C_6H_{10}OH$	50	235	75	350	
2-Methylcyclohexanone	$CH_3CHCO(CH_2)_3CH_2$	50	230	75	345	Sk
Methylcyclopentadienyl manganese tricarbonyl (as Mn)	*see Tricarbonyl (methylcyclopentadienyl)-manganese*					
2-Methyl-4,6-dinitrophenol	$CH_3C_6H_2(OH)(NO_2)_2$	—	0·2	—	0·6	Sk
4,4'-Methylenebis-(2-chloroaniline) (MBOCA)	*see 2,2'-Dichloro-4,4'-methylenedianiline*					
Methylene chloride	*see Dichloromethane*					
4,4'-Methylenediphenyl diisocyanate (MDI)	*see Part 1 for control limit*					
4,4'-Methylenedianiline	$H_2NC_6H_4CH_2C_6H_4NH_2$	0·1	0·8	0·5	4	
Methyl ethyl ketone (MEK)	*see Butan-2-one*					
Methyl ethyl ketone peroxides (MEKP)	$C_8H_{16}O_4$ or $C_8H_{18}O_6$	0·2	1·5	0·2	1·5	
Methyl formate	$HCOOCH_3$	100	250	150	375	
5-Methylheptan-3-one	$CH_3COCH_2CH_3CHCH_2CH_3$	25	130	—	—	
5-Methylhexan-2-one	$CH_3COCH_2CH_2CH(CH_3)_2$	100	475	150	710	
Methyl iodide	*see Iodomethane*					
Methyl isoamyl ketone	*see 5-Methylhexan-2-one*					
Methyl isobutyl carbinol	*see 4-Methylpentan-2-ol*					
Methyl isobutyl ketone (MIBK)	*see 4-Methylpentan-2-one*					
Methyl isocyanate	*see Part 1 for control limit*					
Methyl mercaptan	*see Methanethiol*					
Methyl methacrylate	$CH_2=C(CH_3)COOCH_3$	100	410	125	510	
Methyl parathion	*see Parathion-methyl (ISO)*					

Substance	Formula	Long-term exposure limit (8-hour TWA value)		Short-term exposure limit (10-minute TWA value)		Notes
		ppm	mg m^{-3}	ppm	mg m^{-3}	
4-Methylpentan-2-ol	$CH_3CHOHCH_2CH(CH_3)_2$	25	100	40	160	Sk
4-Methylpentan-2-one	$(CH_3)_2CHCH_2COCH_3$	100	410	125	510	Sk
4-Methylpent-3-en-2-one	$CH_3COCH=C(CH_3)_2$	25	100	—	—	
4-Methyl-m-phenylene d:isocyanate	see Part 1 for control limit					
2-Methylpropan-1-ol	$(CH_3)_2CHCH_2OH$	50	150	75	225	
2-Methylpropan-2-ol	$(CH_3)_3COH$	100	300	150	450	
Methyl propyl ketone	see Pentan-2-one					
Methyl silicate	see Tetramethyl orthosilicate					
α-Methylstyrene	see 2-Phenylpropene					
Methylstyrenes, all isomers except α-Methylstyrene	$CH_3C_6H_4CH=CH_2$	100	480	150	720	
N-Methyl-N-2,4,6-tetranitro-aniline	$(NO_2)_3C_6N(NO_2)CH_3$	—	1·5	—	3	Sk
Mevinphos (ISO)	$C_7H_{13}O_6P$	0·01	0·1	0·03	0·3	Sk
Mica						
total dust		—	10	—	—	
respirable dust (see Appendix 4)		—	1	—	—	
Molybdenum compounds (as Mo),	Mo					
soluble compounds		—	5	—	10	
insoluble compounds		—	10	—	20	
Morpholine	C_4H_9NO	20	70	30	105	Sk
Naled (ISO)	$C_4H_7Br_2Cl_2O_4P$	—	3	—	6	
Naphthalene	$C_{10}H_8$	10	50	15	75	
1,5-Naphthylene diisocyanate	see Part 1 for control limit					
Nickel	Ni					
Nickel compounds (as Ni),	Ni					
soluble compounds		—	0·1	—	0·3	
insoluble compounds		—	1	—	3	

Nickel carbonyl	*see Tetracarbonylnickel*					
Nicotine	$C_{10}H_{14}N_2$	—	0·5	—	1·5	Sk
Nitrapyrin	*see 2-Chloro-6-(trichloromethyl) pyridine*					
Nitric acid	HNO_3	2	5	4	10	
Nitric oxide	*see Nitrogen monoxide*					
4-Nitroaniline	$NO_2C_6H_4NH_2$	1	6	2	12	Sk
Nitrobenzene	$C_6H_5NO_2$	1	5	2	10	Sk
Nitrogen dioxide	NO_2	5	9	5	9	
Nitrogen monoxide	NO	25	30	35	45	
Nitrogen trifluoride	NF_3	10	30	15	45	
Nitroglycerine	*see Glycerol trinitrate*					
Nitromethane	CH_3NO_2	100	250	150	375	Sk
2-Nitropropane	$CH_3CH(NO_2)CH_3$	25	90	25	90	
Nitrotoluene, all isomers	$CH_3C_6H_4NO_2$	5	30	10	60	
Non-siliceous mineral dusts, containing <1% quartz						
total dust		—	10	—	—	
respirable dust (see Appendix 4)		—	5	—	—	
Non-siliceous mineral dusts, containing >1% quartz	*see Appendix 4*					
Octachloronaphthalene	$C_{10}Cl_8$	—	0·1	—	0·3	Sk
n-Octane	$CH_3(CH_2)_6CH_3$	300	1450	375	1800	
Oil mist, mineral		—	5	—	10	
Orthophosphoric acid	H_3PO_4	—	1	—	3	
Osmium tetraoxide (as Os)	OsO_4	0·0002	0·002	0·0006	0·006	
Oxalic acid	$COOHCOOH$	—	1	—	2	
Oxalonitrile	$(CN)_2$	10	20	—	—	
Ozone	O_3	0·1	0·2	0·3	0·6	
PCBs	*see Chlorinated biphenyls*					
Paraffin wax, fume		—	2	—	6	
Paraquat dichloride (ISO), respirable dust (see Appendix 4)	$[CH_3(C_5H_4N^+)_2CH_3]\ 2Cl^-$	—	0·1	—	—	
Parathion (ISO)	$(C_2H_5O)_2PSOC_6H_4NO_2$	—	0·1	—	0·3	Sk

Substance	Formula	Long-term exposure limit (8-hour TWA value)		Short-term exposure limit (10-minute TWA value)		Notes
		ppm	mg m^{-3}	ppm	mg m^{-3}	
Parathion-methyl (ISO)	$C_8H_{10}NO_5PS$	—	0·2	—	0·6	Sk
Pentacarbonyliron (as Fe)	$Fe(CO)_5$	0·01	0·08	—	—	
Pentachlorophenol	C_6Cl_5OH	—	0·5	—	1·5	Sk
Pentaerythritol	$C(CH_2OH)_4$	—	10	—	20	
Pentane, all isomers	C_5H_{12}	600	1800	750	2250	
Pentan-2-one	$CH_3COC_3H_7$	200	700	250	875	
Pentan-3-one	$C_2H_5COC_2H_5$	200	700	250	875	
Pentyl acetate	$CH_3COOC_5H_{11}$	100	530	150	800	
Perchloroethylene	*see Tetrachloroethylene*					
Perchloryl fluoride	ClO_3F	3	14	6	28	
Phenacyl chloride	*see 2-Chloroacetophenone*					
Phenol	C_6H_5OH	5	19	10	38	Sk
p-Phenylenediamine	$C_6H_4(NH_2)_2$	—	0·1	—	—	Sk
Phenylethylene	*see Styrene*					
Phenylhydrazine	$C_6H_5NHNH_2$	5	20	10	45	Sk
2-Phenylpropene	$C_6H_5C(CH_3)=CH_2$	100	480	100	480	
Phorate (ISO)	$C_7H_{17}O_2PS_3$	—	0·05	—	0·2	Sk
Phosdrin	*see Mevinphos (ISO)*					
Phosgene	$COCl_2$	0·1	0·4	—	—	
Phosphine	PH_3	0·3	0·4	1	1	
Phosphorus, yellow	P_4	—	0·1	—	0·3	
Phosphorus pentachloride	PCl_5	0·1	1	—	—	
Phosphorus pentasulfide	*see Diphosphorus pentasulphide*					
Phosphoryl trichloride	$POCl_3$	0·5	3	—	—	
Phthalic anhydride	$C_6H_4(CO)_2O$	1	6	4	24	
Picloram (ISO)	$C_6H_3Cl_3N_2O_2$	—	10	—	20	
Picric acid	$HOC_6H_2(NO_2)_3$	—	0·1	—	0·3	Sk
Platinum salts, soluble (as Pt)	Pt	—	0·002	—	—	
Polychlorinated biphenyls (PCBs)	*see Chlorinated biphenyls*					

Polyvinyl chloride (PVC)						
total dust		—	10	—	—	
respirable dust (see Appendix 4)		—	5	—	—	
Potassium hydroxide	KOH	—	2	—	—	
n-Propanol	see Propan-1-ol					
Propan-1-ol	CH₃CH₂CH₂OH	200	500	250	625	Sk
Propan-2-ol	(CH₃)₂CHOH	400	980	500	1225	Sk
Propargyl alcohol	see Prop-2-yn-1-ol					
Propionic acid	CH₃CH₂COOH	10	30	15	45	
Propoxur (ISO)	H₃CNHCOOC₆H₄OCH(CH₃)₂	—	0·5	—	2	
n-Propyl acetate	CH₃COOC₃H₇	200	840	250	1050	
Propylene dinitrate	CH₃CHONO₂CH₂ONO₂	0·2	2	0·2	2	Sk
Propylene glycol dinitrate (PGDN)	see Propylene dinitrate					
Propylene glycol monomethyl ether	see 1-Methoxypropan-2-ol					
Propylene oxide	see 1,2-Epoxypropane					
Prop-2-yn-1-ol	HC≡CCH₂OH	1	2	3	6	Sk
Pyrethrins (ISO)		—	5	—	10	
Pyridine	C₅H₅N	5	15	10	30	
2-Pyridylamine	NH₂C₅H₄N	0·5	2	2	4	
Pyrocatechol	C₆H₄(OH)₂	5	20	—	—	
Quartz, crystalline						
total dust	SiO₂	—	0·3	—	—	
respirable dust (see Appendix 4)		—	0·1	—	—	
Quinone	see p-Benzoquinone					
RDX	see 1,3,5-Trinitro-1,3,5-triazinane					
Resorcinol	C₆H₄(OH)₂	10	45	20	90	
Rhodium (as Rh),	Rh					
metal fume and dusts		—	0·1	—	0·3	
soluble salts		—	0·001	—	0·003	
Ronnel	see Fenchlorphos (ISO)					
Rosin core solder pyrolysis products						
(as formaldehyde)		—	0·1	—	0·3	
Rotenone (ISO)	C₂₃H₂₂O₆	—	5	—	10	

Substance	Formula	Long-term exposure limit (8-hour TWA value)		Short-term exposure limit (10-minute TWA value)		Notes
		ppm	mg m^{-3}	ppm	mg m^{-3}	
Selenium and compounds, except hexafluoride, (as Se)	Se	—	0·2	—	—	
Selenium hexafluoride (as Se)	SeF$_6$	0·05	0·2	—	—	
Silane	SiH$_4$	0·5	0·7	1	1·5	
Silica, amorphous	SiO$_2$					
total dust		—	6	—	—	
respirable dust (see Appendix 4)		—	3	—	—	
Silica, fused	SiO$_2$					
total dust		—	0·3	—	—	
respirable dust (see Appendix 4)		—	0·1	—	—	
Silicon tetrahydride	see Silane					
Silver	Ag	—	0·1	—	—	
Silver, soluble compounds (as Ag)	Ag	—	0·01	—	0·03	
Sodium azide	Na$_3$N	0·1	0·3	0·1	0·3	
Sodium 2-(2,4-dichloro-phenoxy) ethyl sulphate	C$_8$H$_7$Cl$_2$NaO$_5$S	—	10	—	20	Sk
Sodium fluoroacetate	CH$_2$FCOONa	—	0·05	—	0·15	
Sodium hydrogen sulphite	NaHSO$_3$	—	5	—		
Sodium hydroxide	NaOH	—	2	—	2	
Sodium metabisulphite	see Disodium disulphite					
Stibine	SbH$_3$	0·1	0·5	0·3	1·5	
Strychnine	C$_{21}$H$_{22}$N$_2$O$_2$	—	0·15	—	0·45	
Styrene	C$_6$H$_5$CH=CH$_2$ see Part 1 for new control limit	100	420	125	525	until 31.3.84
Subtilisins (Proteolytic enzymes as 100% pure crystalline enzyme)		—	0·00006	—	0·00006	
Sucrose	C$_{12}$H$_{22}$O$_{11}$	—	10	—	20	
Sulfotep (ISO)	(C$_2$H$_5$)$_4$P$_2$S$_2$O$_5$	—	0·2	—	0·6	
Sulphur dioxide	SO$_2$	2	5	5	13	
Sulphur hexafluoride	SF$_6$	1000	6000	1250	7500	Sk

Substance	Formula / Reference					
Sulphuric acid	H_2SO_4	—	1	—	—	
Sulphur monochloride	*see Disulphur dichloride*					
Sulphur pentafluoride	*see Disulphur decafluoride*					
Sulphur tetrafluoride	SF_4	0·1	0·4	0·3	1	
Sulphuryl difluoride	SO_2F_2	5	20	10	40	Sk
2,4,5-T (ISO)	$C_8H_5Cl_3O_3$	—	10	—	20	
TEDP	*see Sulfotep (ISO)*					
TEPP (ISO)	$(C_2H_5)_4P_2O_7$	0·004	0·05	0·01	0·2	Sk
TNT	*see 2,4,6-Trinitrotoluene*					
Talc total dust		—	10	—	—	
respirable dust (see Appendix 4)		—	1	—	—	
Tantalum	Ta	—	5	—	10	
Tellurium & compounds, except hexafluoride, (as Te)	Te	—	0·1	—	—	
Tellurium hexafluoride (as Te)	TeF_6	0·02	0·2	—	—	
Terphenyls, all isomers	$C_{18}H_{14}$	0·5	5	0·5	5	
Tetrabromomethane	*see Carbon tetrabromide*					
Tetracarbonylnickel (as Ni)	$Ni(CO)_4$	0·05	0·35	—	—	
Tetrachloroethylene	$CCl_2{=}CCl_2$	100	670	150	1000	
Tetrachloromethane	*see Carbon tetrachloride*					
Tetrachloronaphthalenes, all isomers	$C_{10}H_4Cl_4$	—	2	—	4	
O,O,O',O'-Tetraethyl dithiopyrophosphate	*see Sulfotep (ISO)*					
O,O,O',O'-Tetraethyl pyrophosphate	*see TEPP (ISO)*					
Tetraethyl orthosilicate	$Si(OC_2H_5)_4$	10	85	30	255	
Tetrafluorodichloroethane	*see 1,2-Dichlorotetrafluoroethane*					
Tetrahydrofuran	$(C_2H_4)_2O$	200	590	250	735	
Tetramethyl orthosilicate	$(CH_3O)_4Si$	5	30	5	30	
Tetramethyl succinonitrile	$C_8H_{12}N_2$	0·5	3	2	9	Sk
Tetrasodium pyrophosphate	$Na_4P_2O_7$	—	5	—	—	
Tetryl	*see N-Methyl-N 2,4,6-tetranitroaniline*					
Thallium, soluble compounds (as Tl)	Tl	—	0·1	—	—	Sk
4,4'-Thiobis(6-tert-butyl-m-cresol)	*see 6,6'-Di-tert-butyl-4,4'-thiodi-m-cresol*					
Thioglycollic acid	*see Mercaptoacetic acid*					
Thiram (ISO)	$(CH_3)_2NCS_2S_2N(CH_3)_2$	—	5	—	10	
Tin compounds, inorganic, except SnH_4, (as Sn)	Sn	—	2	—	4	

Substance	Formula	Long-term exposure limit (8-hour TWA value)		Short-term exposure limit (10-minute TWA value)		Notes
		ppm	$mg\ m^{-3}$	ppm	$mg\ m^{-3}$	
Tin compounds, organic, except Cyhexatin (ISO), (as Sn)	Sn	—	0·1	—	0·2	Sk
Toluene	$C_6H_5CH_3$	100	375	150	560	Sk
Toluene di-isocyanate (TDI)	see Part 1 for control limit					
o-Toluidine	$CH_3C_6H_4NH_2$	5	22	10	44	
1,4,7-Tri-(aza)-heptane	see 2,2'-Iminodi(ethylamine)					
Tribromomethane	see Bromoform					
Tributyl phosphate, all isomers	$(C_4H_9)_3PO_4$	—	5	—	5	
Tricarbonyl(eta-cyclopentadienyl) manganese (as Mn)	C_5H_5—$Mn(CO)_3$	—	0·1	—	0·3	Sk
Tricarbonyl(methylcyclo-pentadienyl) manganese (as Mn)	$(CH_3)C_5$—$Mn(CO_3)$	—	0·2	—	0·6	Sk
Trichloroacetic acid	CCl_3COOH	1	5	—	—	
1,1,1-Trichlorobis(chlorophenyl)-ethane	$C_{14}H_9Cl_5$	—	1	—	3	
1,1,1-Trichloroethane	CH_3CCl_3	350	1900	450	2450	Sk
1,1,2-Trichloroethane	$CH_2ClCHCl_2$	10	45	20	90	Sk
Trichloroethylene	see Part 1 for control limit					
Trichlorofluoromethane	CCl_3F	1000	5600	1250	7000	
Trichloromethane	see Chloroform					
Trichloronitromethane	CCl_3NO_2	0·1	0·7	0·3	2	
2,4,5-Trichlorophenoxy-acetic acid	see 2,4,5-T (ISO)					
1,2,3-Trichloropropane	$CH_2ClCHClCH_2Cl$	50	300	75	450	
1,1,2-Trichlorotrifluoro-ethane	CCl_2FCClF_2	1000	7600	1250	9500	
Tri-o-cresyl phosphate	see Tri-o-toyl phosphate					
Tricyclohexyltin hydroxide	see Cyhexatin (ISO)					

Substance	Formula					
Tridymite	SiO₂					
total dust		—	0·15	—	—	
respirable dust (see Appendix 4)		—	0·05	—	—	
Triethylamine	(C₂H₅)₃N	25	100	40	160	
Trifluorobromomethane	*see Bromotrifluoromethane*					
Trimanganese tetraoxide	Mn₃O₄	—	1	—	—	
Trimellitic anhydride	*see Benzene-1,2,4-tricarboxylic acid 1,2-anhydride*					
Trimethylbenzenes, all isomers	(CH₃)₃C₆H₃	25	125	35	170	
2,5,5-Trimethylcyclo-hex-2-enone	C₉H₁₄O	5	25	5	25	
2,4,6-Trinitrophenol	*see Picric acid*					
2,4,6-Trinitrotoluene	CH₃C₆H₂(NO₂)₃	—	0·5	—	0·5	
1,3,5-Trinitro-1,3,5-triazinane	C₃H₆N₆O₆	—	1·5	—	3	
Triphenyl phosphate	(C₆H₅)₃PO₄	—	3	—	6	Sk
Tripoli						
total dust		—	0·3	—	—	
respirable dust (see Appendix 4)		—	0·1	—	—	
Tri-o-tolyl phosphate	(CH₃C₆H₄O)₃P=O	—	0·1	—	0·3	
Tungsten & compounds (as W),	W					
soluble		—	1	—	3	
insoluble		—	5	—	10	
Turpentine	~C₁₀H₁₆	100	560	150	840	
Uranium compounds, natural, soluble (as U)	U	—	0·2	—	0·6	
Vanadium pentoxide	*see Divanadium pentaoxide*					
Vinyl acetate	CH₃COOCH=CH₂	10	30	20	60	
Vinyl benzene	*see Styrene*					
Vinyl bromide	*see Bromoethylene*					
Vinyl chloride	*see Part 1 for control limit*					
4-Vinylcyclohexene dioxide	*see 1,2-Epoxy-4-epoxyethylcyclohexane*					
Vinylidene chloride	*see 1,1-Dichloroethylene*					
Vinyltoluenes, all isomers	*see Methylstyrenes, all isomers*					

Substance	Formula	Long-term exposure limit (8-hour TWA value)		Short-term exposure limit (10-minute TWA value)		Notes
		ppm	mg m⁻³	ppm	mg m⁻³	
Warfarin (ISO)	$C_{19}H_{16}O_4$	—	0·1	—	0·3	
Welding fume		—	5	—	—	
White spirit		100	575	125	720	
Wood dust, non-allergenic		—	5	—	10	
Xylene, all isomers	$C_6H_4(CH_3)_2$	100	435	150	650	Sk
Xylidine, all isomers	$(CH_3)_2C_6H_3NH_2$	5	25	10	50	Sk
Yttrium	Y	—	1	—	3	3
Zinc chloride, fume	$ZnCl_2$	—	1	—	2	
Zinc distearate	$Zn(C_{18}H_{35}O_2)_2$	—	10	—	20	
Zinc oxide, fume	ZnO	—	5	—	10	
Zirconium compounds (as Zr)	Zr	—	5	—	10	

Appendix 1. Calculation of 8-hour Time-weighted Averages

(a) Calculation of 8-hour time-weighted averages from full shift samples

Results should normally be reported as an 8-hour time-weighted average. If *one* whole shift sample is taken then the results should be calculated as follows:

(i) if the working shift is exactly 8 hours, then the result of a whole shift sample is the 8-hour time-weighted average;

(ii) if the working shift is less than 8 hours, then the time-weighted average can be calculated assuming zero exposure during the remaining time;

Example
Operator works 7 hr 20 min on a process emitting a substance during shift. Exposure measured at 0.12 mg m^{-3}.
8-hour time-weighted average is computed from:

7 h 20 min (7.33 hr) at 0.12 mg m^{-3}
  40 min (0.67 hr) at 0.00 mg m^{-3}

$$\text{8-hour time-weighted average} = \frac{0.12 \times 7.33}{8}$$

$$= 0.11 \text{ mg m}^{-3}$$

(iii) if the working shift is more than 8 hours then a time-weighted average should be determined for a representative 8-hour period of the working shift.
If the exposure to a substance over the working week is for a period in excess of 40 hours then cognisance should be taken of this when interpreting the results. Care will be needed and such interpretation should be carried out by an experienced occupational hygienist. The following example is given as a guideline for the interpretation of results when an operator has been exposed to the substance for a 50-hour working week. It illustrates the 8-hour time-weighted average being increased on a *pro rata* basis for comparison with the exposure limit.

Example
Operator works 10-hour shift for 5 days
Analysis of 8-hour shift sample shows exposure of 0.07 mg m^{-3}
Man works 50 hours per week. As a guideline for interpretation, the 8-hour time-weighted average is increased *pro rata*.

$$0.07 \times \frac{50}{40} = 0.088 \text{ mg m}^{-3}$$

(b) Calculation of 8-hour time-weighted averages from split samples

Example

Working period	Sampling result (mg m^{-3})	Duration of sampling (hr)
8.00–10.30	0.12	2.5
10.45–12.45	0.07	2
13.30–15.30	0.20	2
15.45–17.15	0.10	1.5

8-hour time-weighted average

$$= \frac{2 \cdot 5(0 \cdot 12) + 2(0 \cdot 07) + 2(0 \cdot 20) + 1 \cdot 5(0 \cdot 10)}{8}$$

$$= \frac{0 \cdot 30 + 0 \cdot 14 + 0 \cdot 40 + 0 \cdot 15}{8}$$

$$= 0 \cdot 12 \text{ mg m}^{-3}$$

The individual period results indicate high exposure during one working period (13·30 to 15·30); this should be investigated for possible changes in working patterns or processes and corrective action taken if the substance has a short-term exposure limit of less than 0·2 mg m^{-3}. This valuable information would not have been apparent from full shift sampling.

(c) Calculation of time-weighted averages for intermittent exposures and their interpretation
The operator's daily working pattern should be known. The exposure level for each job should be measured or estimated from other information.

Example
General labourer/cleaner carried out a variety of tasks over the whole day with exposure levels measured or estimated for each task.

Task	Airborne concentration of substances during task (mg m^{-3})	Normal daily pattern of work (h)
Helping in workshop	0·10 (known to be exposure of full-time group in workshop)	2
Cleaning elsewhere in factory	0 (assumed)	1
Gardening	0 (assumed)	3
Cleaning-up after breakdowns in workshop	0·21 (measured)	2

Likely 8-hour time-weighted average

$$= \frac{2(0 \cdot 10) + 2(0 \cdot 21)}{8}$$

$$= 0 \cdot 078 \text{ mg m}^{-3}$$

Appendix 2. Lead

The control limits for lead are as set out in Appendix 1 of the Health and Safety Commission Approved Code of Practice[7] supporting the Control of Lead at Work Regulations 1980. This Appendix is reproduced below.

The Lead-in-air Standard

1. The standard for lead-in-air is an 8-hour time-weighted average concentration:

Lead, except for tetraethyl lead	(as Pb) 0.15 mg m^{-3} of air
Tetraethyl lead	(as Pb) 0.15 mg m^{-3} of air

When determining lead-in-air concentrations for comparison with the standard, appropriate methods as published by HSE, or other methods which have standards of accuracy equivalent to or better than those methods, should be used.

2. As the extent of lead absorption is related not only to the amount of lead present but also to factors such as composition, solubility, particle size and period of exposure, some departure from the lead-in-air standard may be allowed for the purposes of Regulations 6 (Control Measures for Material, Plant and Processes) and 7 (Respiratory Protective Equipment) provided that:

(a) there is sufficient information available from biological test results to indicate that the degree of lead absorption is at an acceptable level;

(b) 8-hour time-weighted average concentrations do not exceed 3 times the standard set out in para 1.

To be valid for this purpose, the biological tests should have been carried out in persons who do not wear respiratory protective equipment at work, are regularly employed in the workplace and work a standard week in that workplace. Evaluation of lead-in-air results and biological test results in relation to working conditions should be made by an occupational hygienist or other competent person.

Appendix 3. Vinyl Chloride (Chloroethylene)

The control limit is 3 ppm averaged over one year as measured either continuously or by permanent sequential means.[8] Where discontinuous measurements are made, results should be such that it is possible to state with a confidence coefficient of at least 95% that the true mean annual concentration did not exceed 3 ppm.

Table 1 gives guidance on exposure levels for periods of less than one year for control purposes.

These levels must have a maximum 5% probability of being exceeded when the annual arithmetic mean of atmospheric vinyl chloride concentrations is three ppm.

Table 1. Exposure levels for periods of less than one year

Reference period	Limit value in parts per million (rounded off)
One month	5
One week	6
Eight hours	7
One hour	8

Appendix 4. Airborne Dusts

The occupational exposure limits for many dusts are set out in the lists of control and recommended limits. This appendix deals with mixtures and certain specific dusts.

Silica
For mineral dusts containing crystalline silica, the following formulae should be used for the calculation of recommended limits:

Total dust, respirable* & non-respirable

$$= \frac{30}{\% \text{ quartz} + 3} \text{ mg m}^{-3} \text{ 8-hour TWA}$$

Respirable dust*

$$= \frac{10}{\% \text{ respirable quartz} + 2} \text{ mg m}^{-3} \text{ 8-hour TWA}$$

For mineral dusts containing cristobalite or tridymite one half of the value calculated from the above formulae should be used.

Coal Dust
Permitted levels of respirable dust in coal mines are laid down in the Coal Mines (Respirable Dust) Regulations 1975 and the Coal Mines (Respirable Dust Amendment) Regulations 1978.

For coal dust, in workplaces other than coal mines, containing more than 5% quartz the formulae for mineral dust containing crystalline silica should be used.

Graphite
For natural or synthetic graphite containing more than 1% quartz, the formulae for mineral dusts containing crystalline silica should be used.

Cotton
The recommended limit for cotton is $0 \cdot 5$ mg m^{-3} total dust less fly 8-hour TWA using static samplers.[11] This recommended limit is to be applied to the preparatory stages of spinning raw cotton up and including winding and beaming (see Guidance Note EH 25 *Cotton dust sampling*).

References

1 Health and Safety Executive *Pre-employment health screening* Guidance Note MS 20 1982. Available from HMSO.

2 Health and Safety Executive *Health surveillance by routine procedures* Guidance Note MS 18 1981. Available from HMSO.

3 Health and Safety Executive *Isocyanates — medical surveillance* Guidance Note MS 8 1977. Available from HMSO.

* For the purposes of this Guidance Note, respirable dust and total dust are those fractions of the airborne dust which will be collected when sampling is undertaken in accordance with the methods described in MDHS 14 *General methods for the gravimetric determination of respirable and total dust* published by HSE[10].

4 Health and Safety Executive *Styrene* Toxicology Review 1 1981. Available from HMSO.

Health and Safety Executive *Formaldehyde* Toxicology Review 2 1981. Available from HMSO.

Health and Safety Executive *Carbon disulphide* Toxicology Review 3 1981. Available from HMSO.

Health and Safety Executive *Benzene* Toxicology Review 4 1982. Available from HMSO.

Health and Safety Executive *Pentachlorophenol* Toxicology Review 5 1982. Available from HMSO.

Health and Safety Executive *Trichloroethylene* Toxicology Review 6 1982. Available from HMSO.

Health and Safety Executive *Cadmium* Toxicology Review 7 1983. Available from HMSO.

5 Toxikologisch — Arbeitsmedicinische Begrundungen von MAK-Werten. Verlag Chemie, D-6940 Weinhem/Bergstr.

6 ACGIH *Documentation of threshold limit values for substances in workroom air 1982* Available from American Conference of Government Industrial Hygienists, POB 1937, Cincinnati, Ohio 45201.

7 Health and Safety Commission *Control of lead at work* Approved Code of Practice 1980. Available from HMSO.

8 EC Directive 78/610/EEC *Vinyl chloride monomer*.

9 Health and Safety Executive *Asbestos: control limits and measurement of airborne dust concentrations* Guidance Note EH 10.

10 Health and Safety Executive *General method for the gravimetric determination of respirable and total dust* MDHS 14 Available from HMSO.

11 Health and Safety Executive *Cotton dust sampling* Guidance Note EH 25 1981. Available from HMSO.

HSE Publications

Methods for the Determination of Hazardous Substances

MDHS 1 Acrylonitrile in air
Laboratory method using charcoal adsorption tubes and gas chromatography

MDHS 2 Acrylonitrile in air
Laboratory method using porous polymer adsorption tubes, and thermal desorption with gas chromatographic analysis

MDHS 3 Generation of test atmospheres of organic vapours by the syringe injection technique
Portable apparatus for laboratory and field use

MDHS 4 Generation of test atmospheres of organic vapours by the permeation tube method
Apparatus for laboratory use

MDHS 5 On-site validation of sampling methods

MDHS 6 Lead and inorganic compounds of lead in air
Laboratory method using atomic absorption spectrometry

MDHS 7 Lead and inorganic compounds of lead in air
Laboratory method using X-ray fluorescence spectrometry

MDHS 8 Lead and inorganic compounds of lead in air
Colorimetric field method using sym-diphenylthio-carbazone (dithizone)

MDHS 9 Tetra alkyl lead compounds in air
Personal monitoring method

MDHS 10 Cadmium and inorganic compounds of cadmium in air
Laboratory method using atomic absorption spectrometry

MDHS 11 Cadmium and inorganic compounds of cadmium in air
Laboratory method using X-ray fluorescence spectrometry

MDHS 12 Chromium and inorganic compounds of chromium in air
Laboratory method using atomic absorption spectrometry

MDHS 13 Chromium and inorganic compounds of chromium in air
Laboratory method using X-ray fluorescence spectrometry

MDHS 14   General method for the gravimetric determination of respirable and total dust

MDHS 15   Carbon disulphide

MDHS 16   Mercury vapour in air
Laboratory method using hopcalite absorbent tubes, and acid dissolution with cold vapour atomic absorption spectrometric analysis

MDHS 17   Benzene in air
Laboratory method using charcoal adsorbent tubes, solvent desorption and gas chromatography

MDHS 18   Tetra alkyl lead compounds in air
Continuous on-site monitoring method using atomic absorption spectrometry

MDHS 19   Formaldehyde in air
Colorimetric field method using 4,5-dihydroxy-2,7-naphthalenedisulphonic acid

MDHS 20   Styrene in air
Laboratory method using charcoal adsorbent tubes, solvent desorption and gas chromatography

MDHS 21   Glycol ether and glycol ether vapours in air
Laboratory method using charcoal adsorbent tubes, solvent desorption and gas chromatography

MDHS 22   Benzene in air
Laboratory method using porous polymer adsorbent tubes, thermal desorption and gas chromatography

MDHS 23   Glycol ether and glycol ether vapours in air
Laboratory method using Tenax adsorbent tubes, thermal desorption and gas chromatography

MDHS 24   Vinyl chloride in air
Laboratory method using charcoal adsorbent tubes, solvent desorption and gas chromatography

MDHS 25   Organic isocyanates in air
Laboratory method using 1-(2-methoxyphenyl) piperazine solution and high performance liquid chromatography

MDHS 26   Ethylene oxide in air
Laboratory method using charcoal adsorbent tubes, solvent desorption and gas chromatography

MDHS 27   Protocol for assessing the performance of a diffusive sampler

MDHS 28   Chlorinated hydrocarbon solvent vapours in air
Laboratory method using charcoal adsorbent tubes, solvent desorption and gas chromatography

MDHS 29   Beryllium and inorganic compounds of beryllium in air
Laboratory method using atomic absorption spectrometry

MDHS 30   Cobalt and inorganic compounds of cobalt in air
Laboratory method using atomic absorption spectrometry

MDHS 31   Styrene in air
Laboratory method using porous polymer adsorbent tubes, thermal desorption and gas chromatography

MDHS 32   Dioctyl phthalates in air
Laboratory method using Tenax adsorbent tubes, solvent desorption and gas chromatography

MDHS 33   Adsorbent tube standards
Preparation by the syringe loading technique

MDHS 34   Arsine in air
Colorimetric field method using silver diethyldithio-carbamate in the presence of excess silver nitrate.

MDHS 35   Hydrogen fluoride and inorganic fluorides in air
            Laboratory method using an ion selective electrode

Carcinogenesis

A carcinogen is a substance which, administered by any route, increases the incidence of neoplasms in animals or man.

Some industrial toxins are carcinogenic. Identification of a carcinogenic hazard is often delayed because of a long latent period between exposure and the development of clinical symptoms. There are three methods of identifying carcinogens.

1. Epidemiology. Since man began to influence his natural environment, many substances which he has introduced have been found to cause cancer. The widespread use of coal in the 18th century required the employment of chimney sweeps. In 1775 Percival Pott noticed the occurrence of scrotal cancer in these men. Since then many other occupational cancers have been found.

This method of detection is slow, especially if there is a long latent period. It may also be very difficult to establish a causal relationship when the tumour is common in the general population. Accurate occupational histories and long-term follow-up needed.

Newhouse (1965) verified the connection between asbestos and mesothelioma by the study of detailed case histories linked with post-mortem reports at the London Hospital. Plotting of the mesothelioma cases on a map of East London, she was able to show clustering around sites where there had been asbestos factories.

To sharpen epidemiological techniques detailed data collection is needed on an industry-wide, national, or even international scale.

2. Animal Experimentation. By choosing an animal with a short life-span results may be obtained within 1–3 years. Whilst this method has the advantage of more rapid results, it has some disadvantages. The results of animal tests have to be extrapolated to man, and different species have different metabolic systems. For example, α-naphthylamine is not carcinogenic in rats and mice; only man and dog have the glucuronidase enzyme which splits the conjugate and releases the active base in the urinary tract.

3. Short-term Tests. With the proliferation of new chemicals there is an ever-increasing need for some rapid screening for carcinogenicity, and some short-term tests have been developed. These are done in vivo, as implants into experimental animals; in vitro, by studying cell transformation in tissue cultures or the mutation of incubated strains of salmonella (Ames test); and by host-mediated assay in which the test substance is subjected to metabolism, either in vivo or in vitro by incubation with microsomal fractions. Bacterial mutagenicity can be used as a short-term test for chemical carcinogenicity.

All these tests have varying predictability. They are used to set priorities for longer-term conventional animal studies.

Treatment of Intoxication

Although this text is not concerned with treatment, the general principles are mentioned to add emphasis to the need for prevention.

After removal from the source, and decontamination, the treatment methods available are:

1. General supportive and symptomatic treatment.

2. Specific antidotes or chelation.

3. Assisted elimination of the toxin by forced diuresis, peritoneal dialysis, haemodialysis or haemoperfusion.

4. Replacement blood transfusion.

5. Organ transplantation.

Tissue-binding delays excretion. Some toxins, e.g. paraquat, form stable compounds and irreversible changes have occurred by the time the first symptoms appear.

Chelation (Gr. *chele*, a claw). Chelating substances inactivate certain metallic ions, in solution, by strong binding in a ring structure which is stable and soluble.

1. EDTA or Versenate, useful for: lead, plutonium, vanadium, cadmium and manganese.

2. BAL (British Anti-Lewisite; Dimercaptopropanol). Uses a —SH (sulphydryl) radicle which has an affinity for many metals. Effective for arsenic and mercury poisoning. Dimercaptosuccinic acid is also effective in animal tests with lead and mercury. Less toxic than BAL and can be given parenterally or orally.

3. Penicillamine used for Wilson's disease. Sometimes used for oral treatment of lead poisoning, it has been used for mercury poisoning but its usefulness is debatable. The d-isomer is preferred; it can be given orally.

Control of Occupational Hazards — General Principles

Substitution. Can the hazardous material be replaced by one equally effective but less hazardous? (E.g. other solvents for benzene, other insulating materials for asbestos). If not:

Enclosure. Can the whole process be enclosed? If not:

Local Exhaust Ventilation. Does the process lend itself to the drawing off of dust, fume or vapour by local exhaust ventilation?

If none of these things is practicable, *and only then*, reliance must be placed on personal protection.

For dusts, mists and vapours, this means the *appropriate* respirator.

For dermatitis problems, gloves and other protective clothing.

For noise hazards, ear defenders.

Legge's Aphorisms. Sir Thomas Legge, the first Medical Inspector of Factories, enunciated the following principles on the subject of personal protection of the worker:

Unless and until the employer has done everything — and everything means a good deal — the workman can do next to nothing to protect himself, although he is naturally willing enough to do his share.

If you can bring an influence to bear external to the workman (i.e. one over which he can exercise no control), you will be successful; and if you cannot or do not, you will never be wholly successful.

Practically all industrial lead poisoning is due to the inhalation of dust and fume; and if you stop their inhalation you will stop the poisoning.

All workmen should be told something of the danger of the material with which they come into contact and not be left to find it out for themselves — sometimes at the cost of their lives.

CONTROL OF SUBSTANCES HAZARDOUS TO HEALTH

At the time of writing (1984) the Health and Safety Commission has published draft regulations and draft approved codes of practice on this subject. Consultation may lead to some adjustment of the draft, but it is likely that the general philosophy will eventually be incorporated in a statutory document. The proposals intend to consolidate previous legislation on the control of hazardous substances, to expand the control to protect all persons at work and other persons who may be affected from risk to their health associated with exposure to substances hazardous to health arising out of or in connection with work activities.

Four codes of practice are proposed:

1. A general approved code which will apply to all substances hazardous to health, except where a specific code has been approved for a particular substance or process.

2. Approved code of practice for control of carcinogenic substances. This will apply in addition to the general code and not as a substitution for it.

3. An approved code of practice for the control of vinyl chloride monomer.

4. Approved code of practice on fumigation.

Scope. The regulations will apply, subject to some exceptions, to all substances which are hazardous to health by virtue of being very toxic, toxic, harmful, corrosive, or irritant, and to substantial concentrations in air of dust of any kind. The categories are consistent with the proposals for classification, packaging and labelling of substances which form a basis for identifying hazardous substances.

Application

1. Prohibitions. The regulations will schedule a number of substances which are presently prohibited either completely or in certain circumstances.

2. Assessment. There will be a legal requirement to carry out an assessment before starting work which may involve exposure to a substance hazardous to health. An adequate assessment is intended to identify the nature and degree of risk and thus enable the employer or self-employed person to determine the precautions needed to comply with the other regulations — control measures, monitoring and health surveillance.

3. Control. Control of exposure will be required to be achieved through the selection, use and maintenance of appropriate controls over materials, plant and processes. Only where these are not reasonably practicable will personal protective equipment be considered appropriate as a means of controlling exposure. Adequate control of any substance must have regard to any control limit to which the Health and Safety Commission has approved for that substance (*see* p. 117).

4. Health surveillance. This is an important requirement which will be new to most users of substances hazardous to health. Its objectives are to protect individual employees and groups of employees by early detection of any ill effects they may be suffering from as a result of exposure to substances, and to secure the collection, storage and use of data for the detection of hazards to health and the assessment of the efficacy of control measures.

The level of health surveillance will depend upon the nature and degree of the risk. At its most basic level, every employer will be required to keep a record of each of his employees who is exposed to a substance hazardous to health giving simple personal details. The need for other measures, such as routine inspection or an examination by an appointed doctor, will be determined by the circumstances. With a certain limited number of substances specified in a schedule to the regulations an employment medical adviser or appointed doctor will have the powers to suspend an employee from work which exposes him to a substance hazardous to health or impose conditions on his continuing employment.

Carcinogenic Substances. The approved code of practice on the control of carcinogenic substances explains why carcinogens need special attention and it details precautions which should be taken. It emphasizes the importance of elimination, substitution or total containment of the substance.

The code contains a list of substances to which it will apply. At this stage the list is not definitive; it may well be amended following consultation. At the moment the list is as follows:

Acrylonitrile
*4-Aminobiphenyl and its salts
Benzene
Benzo(a)pyrene
2-Chloromethyl ether and technical
    grade chloromethyl methyl ether
3,3′ Dichlorobenzidine and its salts

Diethyl sulphate

Dimethyl sulphate
1-Naphthylamine and its salts
Nickel and nickel compounds
Soots, tars and unrefined mineral oils
4,4′-Bis-*o*-Toluidine and its salts
    (orthotoluidine)

Aflatoxins
Arsenic and arsenic compounds
*Benzidine and its salts
Beryllium and beryllium compounds
Chromium and low solubility chromium
    compounds
B,B′ Dichlorodiethyl sulphide (mustard
    gas)
3,3′ Dimethoxybenzidine and its salts
    (Dianisidine)
Ethylene oxide
*2-Naphthylamine and its salts
*4-Nitrobiphenyl
o-toluidine

Note: VCM is covered by a separate ACOP under the COSHH Regulations.
* These substances are prohibited in the UK except as minor impurities in some other substances or when the subject of a certificate of exemption from these regulations.
   The Code also applies where persons are exposed or liable to be exposed to substances arising from the following processes, although the causative agents have not been identified:
   Auramine and magenta manufacture
   Boot and shoe manufacture and repair where processes involve exposure to leather dust
   Isopropyl alcohol manufacture by the strong acid process.

The Costs of Complying with the Regulations

The Health and Safety Commission point out that the principles of good occupational hygiene practice on which these regulations and codes are based are already applied by good employers who maintain high standards. The cost to them of complying with these regulations should, therefore, be minimal. Where existing controls are not adequate additional costs will arise in assessing risks and in providing practical improvements in working conditions. Substances which are potentially hazardous to health are present in most work places and the regulations will therefore affect nearly all firms from major chemical manufacturers to the smallest craft workshops. The cost of assessment, monitoring of the work place, health surveillance and record keeping will have to be borne by the employers.

Reference

Newhouse M. L. and Thompson H. (1965) *Br. J. Ind. Med.* **22**, 261.

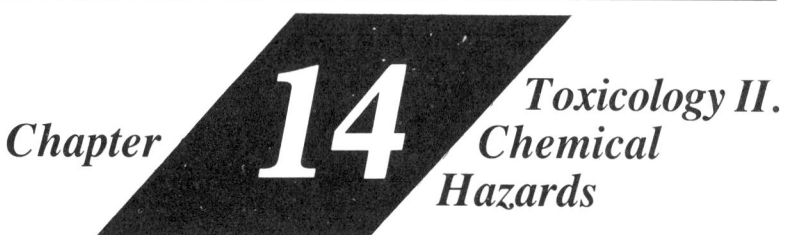

Chapter **14** *Toxicology II. Chemical Hazards*

This section does not purport to be comprehensive, nor to describe in full the toxicology of each material named. It aims to provide a quick source of reference on the main characteristics and toxic effects of each and to serve as a 'signpost' to the standard reference books, a list of which appears in the bibliography at the end of the section.

Treatment of poisoning is not mentioned, except in those few cases where a specific antidote exists. Preventive measures are not stated because they will always include measures to prevent inhalation of dust or fume, and when skin absorption can occur, to avoid skin contamination.

METALS (INCLUDING METALLOIDS)

Aluminium

Metal and its salts not toxic to man. (Absorbed hardly at all from digestive tract.)
Effects of inhalation: thought at one time aluminium dust might have prophylactic action against silicosis and coal workers' pneumoconiosis. Trials disproved this.
Shaver's disease. Interstitial fibrosis of lung observed in abrasives industry in 1947. Exposure was to fumes derived from bauxite fused at 2000 °C; silica, iron and other materials also present, and role of aluminium not known. Condition has not been seen in recent years — but fine aluminium power can cause severe pulmonary fibrosis.

Antimony (Stibium)

TLV 0·5 mg/m^3. Metalloid, similar to arsenic. Forms alloys with lead, tin, zinc, copper and arsenic.
Uses: With lead, in pewter, Britannia metal, printers' type.
Toxicity: Mainly by ingestion — rare in industry. Similar to that of arsenic, but less so. Gastrointestinal and CNS symptoms. Liver poison. BAL (dimercaprol) is specific antidote.

Stibine (SbH$_3$) evolved when antimony compounds meet steam or acids. Highly toxic.
Symptoms: Headache, nausea and vomiting; haematuria; jaundice; anaemia.

Arsenic

TLV Arsenic and compounds $0·2$ mg/m^3; Calcium arsenate $1·0$ mg/m^3; Lead arsenate $0·15$ mg/m^3. Metalloid — intermediate in properties between metal and non-metal: contaminant of commercial acids and many metals.

Uses: In metal alloys, especially copper.

As hardening agent in lead shot.

In rat poison, fungicides, pesticides and weed killers.

As a depilatory in tanning.

Acute poisoning is usually by ingestion and is very rare in industry. Symptoms are nausea, vomiting, diarrhoea, collapse, coma and death.

Chronic poisoning: Peripheral neuritis tending to be sensory rather than motor.

Hepatitis, cirrhosis of the liver and cancers of various sites may occur. The oxide As_2O_3 is not carcinogenic per se, but requires a 'promoter', such as SO_2 or metal oxide fumes.

Keratoses and epitheliomata of skin.

Melanosis.

Antidote: BAL (British Anti-Lewisite; dimercaprol).

Notifiable and prescribed disease.

Biological monitoring of limited value. Tentative criteria for acceptable limits: Blood 50 µg/dl; Urine 1000 µg/dl; Hair 5 ppm; Toenails 10 ppm.

Arsine (Arseniuretted hydrogen, AsH$_3$). TLV $0·05$ ppm. Highly toxic gas smelling of garlic.

Produced when metals containing arsenical impurities (as many do, e.g. copper, lead, zinc, tin, gold) react with acids or by hydrolysis of metallic arsenides, as when calcined metallic ores containing arsenic are quenched with water.

Arsine poisoning usually acute. First sign (as a rule preceded by time lag after exposure) passing of port-wine coloured urine, due to haemoglobinuria. Followed by jaundice, abdominal or back pain, anuria, headache. Massive haemolysis causes haemoglobinuria. Damage to renal tubules and liver may occur.

Chronic poisoning may occur, with anaemia and renal damage.

Prescribed industrial disease under Industrial Injuries Act. Notifiable under Factories Act.

Barium

Soluble salts are toxic when ingested, but there is no hazard to man under industrial conditions. Barium sulphate is insoluble in water, and can safely be swallowed, hence its use as contrast medium in radiography.

Inhaled, it may cause baritosis, a benign pneumoconiosis.

Beryllium

Hard silver-grey metal. SG $1·85$. MP 1280 °C. TLV $0·002$ mg/m^3.

Occurs naturally as beryl (beryllium silicate) which appears to be non-toxic. But metal and its other compounds highly toxic.

Sources of exposure

1. In alloys with copper, nickel, zinc, steel and magnesium. Copper alloys have high tensile strength and high thermal and electrical conductivity. Beryllium bronzes are used for non-spark tools and electrical switchgear.

2. In nuclear reactor research.

3. In the aerospace industry.

4. Melting of non-ferrous scrap or burning.

Hazards: Systemic. Enters body by inhalation, or through cracks and abrasions in skin.

Acute poisoning: Cough and dyspnoea; Irritation of mucous membranes; Acute pneumonitis — may be fatal; Dermatitis; Conjunctivitis; Skin ulcers and granulomata.

Chronic poisoning: Cough and dyspnoea. Time lag 15–20 years. Joint pains; Loss of weight; X-ray appearances of beryllium granulomatosis mimic those of sarcoidosis; may also be confused with miliary TB or silicosis. Relentlessly progressive. Berylliosis has been shown to be due to a cell-damaging reaction between Be antigen and antibody.

Pre-employment screening: Chest X-ray advisable. Lung function tests. Exclusion of those with history of asthma or eczema advised.

Periodic examination: Chest X-ray (annual). Lung function tests. Continuous recording of body weight.

Cadmium

Soft ductile metal. MP 321 °C. BP 767 °C. TLV 0·05 mg/m^3 (metal), 0·2 mg/m^3 (soluble salts).

Uses

1. In brazing alloys with copper, silver and tin to increase hardness. (Fluoborates of alkali metals used as fluxes.)

2. As anti-rust plating material.

3. As electrode in alkaline storage batteries.

4. Cadmium salts are used as pigments and colouring agents for plastics, ceramics and glass.

5. In nuclear reactors as neutron absorbing material.

Hazards: Mainly from inhalation during heating, soldering, welding or burning of cadmium-coated metal. *No immediate irritant effect or distinctive smell.*

Poisoning: Acute: Like metal fume fever. May progress to chemical pneumonitis. *Chronic:* Dyspnoea (due to emphysema) usually without cough. Proteinuria. Renal damage is indicated by the presence in urine of β_2-microglobulin. Chronic renal failure may follow. Skeletal damage like osteomalacia with pseudo-fractures. Anosmia.

Pre-employment screening: Exclude those with history of renal or chronic respiratory disease.

Periodic examinations: Blood and urinary cadmium estimation. (*Note:* Cadmium may be retained in the body for years — mainly in the liver — and excreted very slowly). Hence blood levels tend to be a more reliable index of recent absorption.

Urinary tests for protein and lung function tests 6 monthly.

Chromium

Chromates are carcinogenic when inhaled in powder form.

Chrome salts are not highly toxic, but in chrome-plating may cause skin ulceration and perforation of nasal septum. Hexavalent salts are more toxic than trivalent.

Chromium Plating Regulations no longer require periodical medical inspection of plating workers. Instead, regular monitoring of chromic acid mist is required in all plating shops.

Cobalt

Usually found in association with nickel and iron. Essential trace element for haemopoiesis in human metabolism. 80% of world output used in metallic state.

In machine-tool industry, cobalt dust may be produced together with that of tungsten carbide. Inhalation can cause a pneumoconiosis known as 'hard metal disease'. Estimation of urinary cobalt is a satisfactory way of monitoring. In unexposed people, less than 3 nmol/mmol creatinine occurs.

Skin and pulmonary sensitization to cobalt salts have been recorded.

Copper

Copper salts are poisonous when ingested, but industrial poisoning rarely occurs.

Copper is, however, one of the metals which can cause *metal fume fever* when fumes produced in welding are inhaled.

Gold

Extensively used in electronics industry, jewellery and dentistry. Little is known of its toxicity, but its salts may cause dermatitis.

Iron

Metal and its salts not toxic to man in industrial conditions.

Inhalation of metallic iron causes a benign pneumoconiosis with radiographic mottling but no apparent effect on lung function (siderosis).

Lead

Metal and its compounds widely used in industry. MP 327 °C, BP 1740 °C. Control limit 0·15 mg/m^3 for 40-hour week.

Previous Regulations under the Factories Acts requiring periodic medical examinations of lead workers did not cover all the industrial processes involving lead and its salts. These have now been superseded by the Control of Lead at Work Regulations, which are described below (p. 157).

Lead poisoning: One of the oldest industrial diseases to be recognized. Notifiable under Factories Act. Prescribed disease under Industrial Injuries Act.

Processes with a lead hazard

Lead battery manufacture.
Smelting and refining of ores containing lead.
Manufacture of lead sheet and lead shot.
Making of alloys with other metals.
Scrap metal recovery.
Pottery industry (lead glazes).
Shipbuilding and shipbreaking.
Demolition of buildings (oxyacetylene burning of paint-covered girders).

Plumbing and soldering.

Manufacture and use of lead-based paints.

Vitreous enamelling.

Lead salts, e.g. chromate ore, used as pigments to give colour in plastics industry.

Lead is a cumulative poison, which is stored in and mobilized from bone in the same way as calcium. It is excreted in faeces and urine. Lead concentrations in the blood can readily be measured, and removal from contact can usually be arranged before levels sufficient to cause overt poisoning are reached. For this reason, it is one of the most satisfactory hazards to control by biological monitoring.

Biochemical and haematological effects: There is interference with haemoglobin synthesis. This may produce:

Raised urinary coproporphyrin and ALA (δ-aminolaevulinic acid).

Hypochromic anaemia with anisocytosis, poikilocytosis and raised reticulocyte count (possibly also haemolysis of red cells).

Punctate basophilia.

Early symptoms of poisoning: Non-specific. Fatigue, lethargy, inability to concentrate.

Anorexia and dyspepsia.

Headache, constipation or intermittent diarrhoea.

Established poisoning showing all the classical features is now rare. These are:

Lead colic. May simulate an abdominal emergency.

Lead palsy. Tends to affect the muscles most frequently used and fatigued.

Lead encephalopathy is now rare.

A blue line on the gums at the gingival margin of the teeth when dental hygiene is poor may still be seen occasionally. Indicative of high exposure, not necessarily of poisoning.

Biological monitoring: Blood lead readings over 3·9 μmol/l (80 μg/dl) are regarded as excessive, and indications for a repetition of the test. Readings over 4·9 μmol/l (100 μg/dl) are normally taken as indication for suspension from lead work. However, clinical judgement must always be exercised, and in borderline cases regard must be had in addition to:

Haemoglobin. A fall below 12 g/dl in a man or 11 g/dl in a woman, coupled with high blood lead, may be grounds for suspension.

Urinary ALA (δ-aminolaevulinic acid) >300 μmol/l.

Free erythrocyte protoporphyrin. The measurement of FEP, or ZPP (zinc protoporphyrin) is used as an indicator of lead exposure. FEP does not immediately increase on first exposure to lead, but does so after a time lag of 2 weeks to 2 months. It can remain high for up to a year after exposure ceases.

In people not exposed to lead, levels are usually less than 14 μg/dl, but high levels are found in iron-deficiency anaemia.

An FEP figure of 100 μg/dl corresponds roughly to a blood lead of 60 μg/dl, and 250 μg/dl to 80 μg/dl.

Chelation: Substances such as disodium versenate (EDTA) may be given to hasten the excretion of lead stored in the bones. The calcium salt is formed, from which lead displaces the calcium, the resulting compound being excreted in the urine.

Without chelation, it may take years to excrete all the lead stored in the skeleton after lengthy exposure. Delayed symptoms of lead poisoning have been encountered from this cause after occupational exposure has ceased.

Organic Lead. Tetra-ethyl lead Control Limit 0·1 mg/m^3.

Absorbed through skin as well as by inhalation.

Toxic effects: On CNS. Insomnia, headaches, excitement, agitation and nightmares → delirium, convulsions, mania and coma.

Blood lead and urinary coproporphyrin estimations are not reliable indicators.

Control of Lead at Work Regulations (S.I. 1980 No. 1248). Along with these Regulations the Health and Safety Executive issued an approved Code of Practice giving practical guidance.

Previous Regulations related to specific processes. These Regulations place upon the employer the onus of assessing the nature and extent of exposure to lead. If this is 'significant' (*see below*), all the Regulations apply, but below this level only some of them.

'Significant' is defined as exposure:

(*a*) to levels of air-borne lead of more than half the lead-in-air standard;

(*b*) to a substantial risk of ingesting lead;

(*c*) to skin contact with concentrated lead alkyls.

The lead-in-air standard is an 8-hour time-weighted average of $0 \cdot 15$ mg/m^3 for inorganic lead and $0 \cdot 10$ mg/m^3 for tetraethyl lead.

Medical surveillance by an employment medical adviser or appointed doctor is required if the lead exposure is significant, or if the EMA or AD believes surveillance to be advisable. This will include blood lead estimations, normally at 3-month intervals, as well as an initial clinical assessment, and a haemoglobin estimation at least once a year. When experience has shown blood lead levels to be regularly under 40 μg/100 ml, the interval between examinations may be extended to 12 months; below 60 μg/100 ml, to 6 months. Any individual showing a blood lead level over 80 μg/100 ml must be suspended from lead work, unless he has had at least 20 years' exposure, or at least 10 years if he is over 40 years of age — in which case his suspension is a matter for the discretion of the EMA or AD. Return to lead work must depend on the decision of the EMA or AD that he may safely do so.

Surveillance of workers exposed to lead alkyls requires periodic estimations of lead in urine, after an initial clinical assessment and blood lead estimation, and blood lead should be estimated annually. If urinary lead is below 120 μg/litre, tests should be performed every 6 weeks, between 120 and 149 weekly, and at the doctor's discretion if the level is over 150. A reading of 150 or over is grounds for suspension from exposure.

The Regulations require the employer to have equipment for monitoring lead-in-air, and to use it; to ensure that employees are given adequate information and training, suitable respiratory equipment and protective clothing, and adequate washing and changing facilities. Eating, drinking and smoking in the work-place are not to be allowed. The work-place must be kept clean, and protective equipment maintained in a clean and efficient condition. Records of air monitoring, medical surveillance and biological tests must be kept, and must be available for inspection by employees (to whom, however, individual health records will not be available).

Manganese

TLV 5 mg/m^3

Uses: In steel industry for making of particular alloys. As dioxide, in manufacture of potassium permanganate, in dry batteries, and for colouring glass.

Absorption: Through lungs as dust or fume.

Toxic effects: On CNS through basal ganglia → Parkinson's syndrome. (Requires very heavy exposure; not now seen in Britain.)

Pneumonitis.

MnO_2 mildly irritant to upper respiratory tract.

Biological tests can be used to measure blood and urinary Mn.

Normal levels: blood 90–270 nmol/l, urine 0·2–3·0 nmol/mmol creatinine.

Manganese poisoning is a notifiable and a prescribed industrial disease.

Mercury

Metallic liquid, BP 357 °C. TLV 0·05 mg/m^3.

Vaporizes at room temperature — hence spillage into crevices of floors and benches may constitute unrecognized inhalation hazard.

Also *absorbed through skin.*

Uses: In electrical and electronic industry — batteries, transformers, mercury vapour lamps.

Scientific instruments.

Making of amalgams for dentistry and other purposes.

Chemical industry.

Toxic effects: Acute: Gastro-enteritis with gingivitis and stomatitis. Acute pneumonitis. Renal damage.

Chronic: Insidious onset — headache, lassitude, anorexia. Erethism — jumpiness, timidity, irritability, loss of concentration. Tremors — hands, eyelids, tongue. Gingivitis. Renal tubular damage. (Mercurialentis, a grey discoloration of anterior capsule of eye lens, indicates absorption but not necessarily poisoning.)

Biological monitoring: Excreted in urine. Diurnal variations in rate of excretion, so that 24-hour specimens give more accurate picture. Blood mercury reflects exposure over previous 7 days. 150 nmol/l corresponds to exposure equal to the Recommended Limit (TLV).

Levels correlate with *exposure*, not poisoning; but if level of 300 µg/l (1500 nmol/l) is exceeded, serious thought should be given to removal from contact even in absence of signs and symptoms.

Notifiable industrial disease.

Prescribed industrial disease.

Organic Mercurials

Aryl salts TLV 0·05 mg/m^3.

Alkyl salts TLV 0·01 mg/m^3.

Used principally in powder form as seed dressings; also as fungicide in paints, and in paper making.

Irritant to skin and mucous membranes.

Alkyl salts toxic to CNS — early effects like erethism, followed by peripheral neuropathy and ataxia. (No record of similar effects with aryl salts.)

Urinary excretion: Much lower levels lead to consideration of removal from contact than those for inorganic mercury, 30 µg/l (150 nmol/l) is suggested as upper limit.

Nickel

Metallic nickel and salts not toxic to man, but can cause dermatitis.

Nickel Carbonyl (Ni(CO)$_6$) however, which is used in separating nickel from other metals, is highly toxic, causing pulmonary oedema coming on some hours after exposure. Death may occur from interstitial pneumonitis.

Continued exposure may cause lung cancer — nickel-refining industry shows greatly increased incidence.

Platinum

Other metals in same group — ruthenium, rhodium, palladium, osmium and iridium. MP 1773·5 °C. TLV 2 µg/m^3.

Platinum is separated from other metals of the group, with which it may occur naturally, by conversion into ammonium or sodium chloroplatinates, from which it is isolated by thermal decomposition as a platinum sponge.

Uses: As catalyst in wide range of chemical processes. Laboratory crucibles and other heat- and corrosion-resisting equipment. As anode in some electrolytic processes. Photographic processes. In jewellery.

Toxicology. Platinum salts are sensitizers, and may produce asthma, dermatitis, rhinitis and conjunctivitis. The metal does not appear to possess these properties, which are mainly found in chloroplatinates. Sensitization is usually permanent.

Because it is believed that atopic individuals are at greater risk of sensitization, skin prick tests with the common allergens are now recommended as part of pre-employment screening, positive reactors being excluded.

Periodic skin tests for sensitization to platinum, using high dilutions of platinum salts, are advised, and workers should be informed of the symptoms and encouraged to report them promptly. (HSE Guidance Note MS 22.)

Note: Ulceration of nasal septum has been reported after exposure to ruthenium salts.

Selenium

TLV 0·05 ppm. Inorganic compounds cause dermatitis. Irritant to skin and mucous membranes.

Hydrogen selenide (H$_2$Se) acutely irritant and toxic — garlic smell on breath. May affect CNS, causing lassitude and dizziness.

Silver

Not known to be toxic to man, but heavy exposure may produce skin pigmentation (argyria) and staining of the conjunctivae.

Strontium

Similar in metabolism to calcium, and apparently non-toxic. Radioactive strontium may be taken up by bones.

Tellurium

Less toxic than selenium. Industrial poisoning rare apart from effects of hydrogen telluride, H_2Te, whose effects are similar to those of hydrogen selenide, but less severe, and which has a similar garlic odour. BAL and ascorbic acid have been tried as antidotes, but their value is not proved.

Thallium

TLV 0.1 mg/m^3. Soft malleable metal found naturally in association with cadmium, zinc, copper, arsenic and antimony.
Uses: Catalyst in many organic reactions. In optical instruments. Insecticide and rodenticide. In low-temperature thermometry (with mercury). In metallic alloys.
Acute poisoning: Rare in industry. Gastrointestinal symptoms; convulsions; pains in joints; proteinuria.
Chronic poisoning: CNS symptoms — fatigue, pains in limbs (peripheral neuritis). Loss of hair.

Thorium

Toxicity very low. It is, however, the parent of a series of radioactive elements, and processes using thorium may be subject to Ionizing Radiation Regulations.

Tin

Metal and its salts not toxic to man in industrial conditions. Inhalation of metallic tin causes a 'benign pneumoconiosis' with radiographic mottling but no apparent effect on lung function (stannosis).

Organic tin compounds are highly irritant, causing erythema, burns and blistering, and are used as fungicides.

Titanium

Titanium tetrachloride is highly toxic and irritant, and can cause skin burns, conjunctivitis and keratitis. It is made as part of the the process of extraction of metallic Ti, and readily hydrolyses to HCl.

Tungsten

Only hazard appears to be hard metal disease, a pneumoconiosis found in machine tool industry where there is exposure to mixed dusts of tungsten carbide and cobalt.

Vanadium

TLV Metal 0.5 mg/m^3. Pentoxide 0.05 mg/m^3.
Sources of exposure: Steel industry — constituent of hard metals. Catalyst in some chemical processes, e.g. cracking of oils, sulphuric acid manufacture. Found in crude oils especially those from Western Hemisphere.

Vanadium pentoxide is irritant, and may be encountered in cleaning oil-fired boilers. Skin and mucous membranes affected. Systemic absorption produces vomiting and diarrhoea and a characteristic dark green tongue. Heavy exposure may affect CNS — drowsiness, tremors, convulsions.

Chronic exposure may cause symptoms of bronchitis and asthma.

Zinc

Uses: Production of galvanized steel. As constituent of brass and bronze. Zinc chloride used as flux in tinning.

The metal is non-toxic, but welding and brazing of brass may cause metal fume fever — a febrile condition with influenza-like symptoms coming on 8–10 hours after exposure and usually passing off within 24 hours. This appears to be an allergic reaction to the oxide. (Copper and cadmium and other metals may also cause metal fume fever.)

Zirconium

Used in iron and other alloys — low toxicity.

Skin contact may cause granulomata. Inhaled dust may cause simple pneumoconiosis.

ORGANIC SOLVENTS

Table 14.1, pp. 162, 163, reproduced with acknowledgements to the Notes of Guidance of the Employment Medical Advisory Service, summarizes some important characteristics of the commonly used organics solvents.

ADDITIONAL NOTES ON SOLVENTS

Benzene (C_6H_6)

Benzene

(Distinguish from benzine, a petroleum derivative — mixture of aliphatic hydrocarbons with straight chain structure.)

Benzol is commercial benzene containing other hydrocarbons.

BP 80·1 °C. TLV 10 ppm. Vapour heavier than air. (In USA, 1 ppm from 21 May 1977.)

Handling nowadays usually in closed systems — distillation of fossil fuels in the chemical industry for the synthesis of many substances, and in the blending of motor fuels.

It is no longer used purely for its solvent properties, since there are many

Table 14.1. Properties of certain commonly encountered organic solvents and liquids (By courtesy of the Health and Safety Executive)

Solvent	Synonyms or Trade names	Principal uses	TLV ppm v/v	Volatility	Narcotic (ψ) and Hazard coding	Possible substitutes
A Benzene	Benzol	Chemical synthesis solvent	25	++++	++++ May also cause chronic intoxication (qv)	Benzene — nitration grade
Toluene	Methyl benzene	Rubber adhesives; Solvent	200	+++	+++	Toluene — nitration grade; Xylene
Xylene	Dimethyl benzene	Solvent: paints	100	++	++	
Styrene	Vinyl benzene: phenylethylene	Polystyrene plastics	100	++	++ Irritant effects prominent	Toluene — nitration grade for Toluene '90'
Naphtha (coal tar)	Solvent naphtha	Powerful solvent e.g. for rubber	100	++	+++	Benzene-free naphtha
Naphtha (petroleum)	White spirit Turps substitute	Paint thinner	500	+	+ Mainly dermatitis	
B Methanol	Methyl alcohol wood spirit	Denaturize ethyl alcohol paint solvent	200	+++	+ (note specific eye effects)	Ethanol or IMS
Ethanol	Ethyl alcohol	Solvent, Organic syntheses	1000	++	±	
Propanol-2	Isopropyl alcohol	Ethanol substitute	400	++		
Cyclohexanol		Cellulose solvent: printing inks	50	+	+	
Ethylene chlorohydrin	Monochloro ethyl alcohol	Cellulose solvent	5	+	++ May cause systemic poisoning	
Diacetone alcohol	—	'Anti-blush' agent in cellulose paints	50	±	+	
C Acetone	Dimethyl ketone	General solvent	1000	++++	±	
Methyl ethyl ketone	MEK	General solvent	200	+++	±	
Methyl butyl ketone	MBK	General solvent	100	++	±	
Cyclohexanone	—	Lacquer solvent printing inks	50	+	±	
D Diethyl ether	'Ether' Diethyl oxide	Solvent	400	++++	±	
Ethylene oxide		Fumigant	50	++++	++ (may cause pulmonary oedema)	
Dichloro ethyl ether		Organic synthesis: wax solvent:	15	±	++ (pulmonary oedema)	
Ethyl glycol monoethyl ether	Cellosolve Oxitol	Cellulose paint solvent	25	±	±	
Diethylene glycol monoethyl ether	Carbitol		NS	±	±	
Dioxan	Diethylene dioxide	Wax, paint and lacquer solvents	100	++	± Renal damage if ingested	
Tetrahydrofuran	—	Resin and lacquer solvent	200	+++	+	

Group	Substance	Alternative name	Uses	TLV	Toxicity	Fire hazard	Remarks
E	Ethyl acetate	—	Paint and lacquer solvent	400	++	±	
	Methyl formate	—	Cellulose solvent: insecticide	100	++	+	
	Amyl acetate		Cellulose solvent	100	+	±	
F	Methyl chloride	Monochloromethane	Refrigerant	100	+++	+	Damage to CNS with chronic exposure
	Methylene chloride	Dichloromethane	Degreaser and paint stripper	500	+++	±	
	Chloroform	Trichloromethane	Solvent	50	++	+	
	Carbon tetrachloride	Tetrachloromethane	Solvent for rubber etc.	10	++	+++	
	Ethyl chloride	Monochloroethane		1000	++++	+	Methyl chloroform
	Ethylene dichloride	Dichloroethane	General solvent for waxes, lacquers	50	++	++	
	Methyl chloroform	1,1,1, Trichloroethane	'Cold' liquid phase and vapour degreaser	350	++	±	
	Tetrachloroethane	Acetylene tetrachloride	Cellulose solvent	5	+	++++	
	Trichloroethylene	Trilene, Triklone	Vapour degreaser	100	++	+	Trichloroethylene, Tetrachloroethylene, Member of Group G
	Tetrachloroethylene	Perchloroethylene, Tetrachloroethylene	Vapour degreaser	100	±	±	
	Vinyl chloride		Refrigerant, PVC synthesis	3(CL)	++++	+	
G	Bromo and/or fluoro substituted methanes and ethanes and chloromethanes and ethanes e.g. Trichloro Trifluoroethane	Arklone P	Aerosols, Non-toxic fire extinguishers, solvents	Most are 1000	++++	− or ±	Trichloroethylene or SBP petroleum mixture
H	Carbon disulphide	—	Cellulose solvent (viscose rayon), Rubber solvent	20	++++	++++	May also cause chronic intoxication (qv)

Notes:

1. *Key to index letters*

A Hydrocarbons	E Esters
B Alcohols	F Chlorohydrocarbons
C Ketones	G Halogenated hydrocarbons other than chlorohydrocarbons
	H Carbon disulphide

2. *Threshold Limit Values* are as published in Technical Data Note No. 2/71-TLV for 1971. The TLV is a level which is related to an eight hour per day exposure. If exceeded continuously toxic or other adverse effects may occur. The *volatility* of the liquid will determine, other factors excluded, how quickly the TLV may be attained.
The hazard rating is an approximate indication of the danger to be anticipated from use of the liquid. It is based on practical experience and takes into account both the inherent toxicity and volatility.

3. *Fire hazard.* This may be considerable and the main factor to take into account but is not included as a factor in assessing the hazard rating in the table. In general, the hydrocarbons, the alcohols, ketones, ethers and esters and acetates and also carbon disulphide was flammable or highly flammable and may form explosive mixtures with air. The simpler chlorohydrocarbons are also flammable, some e.g. ethyl chloride and vinyl chloride highly so. With increasing chlorine substitution, flammability decreases and many solvents in this class are non-flammable, e.g. carbon tetrachloride used in fire extinguishers. The bromo and fluoro substituted hydrocarbons are all non-flammable.

equally effective substitutes; but in the past was used in the rubber industry, and a wide range of other industries as a degreaser.

Benzene is narcotic — 1500 ppm can produce dizziness in a few minutes.

Chronic benzene poisoning may cause: aplastic anaemia by general depressant effect on bone marrow; leukaemia or aleukaemic leukaemia; erythroleukaemia.

Principal metabolite on absorption is phenol. Urinary phenol measurement is a fair index of absorption. After 8 hours exposure to the time-weighted average TLV, phenol level is 100 mg/l. Monitoring of benzene concentrations in blood is also possible.

Thrombocytopenia may give early warning of excessive exposure.

Note: Many commercial solvents may contain benzene as a contaminant, especially toluol.

Benzene poisoning is a notifiable industrial disease and a prescribed industrial disease.

Toluene ($C_6H_5CH_3$)

TLV 100 ppm. Possesses most of the solvent properties of benzene, for which it is therefore often used as a substitute.

Like benzene it has a narcotic effect, but has no toxic effect on bone marrow or the liver. As a fat solvent it may cause dermatitis.

(Commercial toluol and xylol may contain up to 6% of benzene).

Metabolite hippuric acid, excreted in urine — test has been used as index of exposure. Normal levels in non-exposed 100–1000 mg/l. Exposed people produce much higher figures. But blood toluene estimation now possible; 45 μmol/l ≡ 100 ppm in air. (Alcohol intake will cause spuriously high figures.)

Xylene ($C_6H_4(CH_3)_2$)

TLV 100 ppm. Effects of over-exposure similar to those of toluene.

Methyl Alcohol (Methanol, Wood Spirit)

TLV 200 ppm. Widely used as solvent and as ingredient of anti-freeze mixtures.

Powerful narcotic which also has long-term effects on CNS, including optic atrophy and peripheral neuritis. Also irritant, and *absorbed through skin.*

Nowadays industrial poisoning is rare, but poisoning not uncommon in those drinking mixtures containing it for intoxicant effect.

Ketones (contain C=O group)

Names end in '-one'. Those commonly used in industry are acetone, methyl ethyl ketone (MEK) and methyl butyl ketone (MBK).

They are degreasers and solvents, having irritant effects on skin and mucous membranes, but of low toxicity.

Unlikely to cause systemic poisoning because of irritant properties.

Carbon Disulphide (CS_2)

CL 10 ppm. Colourless liquid with characteristic offensive smell.

Uses: Solvent for fats, resins and oils, used in rubber industry and in manufacture of certain man-made fibres.

By-product of coal tar distillation.

Toxic effects: Narcotic. Skin irritant. Chronic exposure causes polyneuritis. Headache, giddiness, weakness. Chronic effects include optic neuritis, Parkinsonism, mania. Has also been shown to predispose to coronary heart disease and cerebral atherosclerosis.

Absorbed through skin.

Notifiable industrial disease.

Methyl Bromide (CH$_3$Br) (Monobromomethane)

TLV 5 ppm, 20 mg/m^3.

Heavy colourless almost odourless gas. Decomposed by heat $\rightarrow$ HBr, CO$_2$ in water.

Uses: In fire extinguishers (now largely abandoned): As refrigerant: Fumigating agent: Laboratory reagent.

Hazards: Highly toxic — onset insidious.

May be inhaled, ingested or *absorbed through skin.*

Can be monitored by estimating total blood bromide (after exclusion of medication as possible source). Limit suggested 2 mg/dl.

Acute poisoning: Lung irritation. Respiratory distress 48 hours after exposure. Headache, diplopia and dizziness; Nausea and vomiting; Burning and blistering of skin.

Treatment: Symptomatic.

Methyl chloride and iodide have similar properties.

Chlorinated Hydrocarbons (see also p. 163)

Highly toxic are: Carbon tetrachloride (CCl$_4$). Liver poison, CNS (*See below*) TLV 10 ppm. Tetrachloroethane (CHCl$_2$ — CHCl$_2$). Liver poison, CNS, TLV 5 ppm. These are now seldom used in industry.

Vinyl chloride, used in PVC synthesis, may cause angiosarcoma of the liver; can also produce acro-osteolysis of digital bones.

Control Limit now 10 ppm (TWA)

The less toxic chlorinated hydrocarbons produce mainly narcotic effects if RL exceeded. Those commonly used as industrial solvents and degreasers include: Trichloroethylene (CHCl=CCl$_2$); Tetrachloroethylene (Perchlorethylene) (CCl$_2$=CCl$_2$); 1,1,1 Trichloroethane (Methyl chloroform) (CH$_3$CCl$_3$); Ethyl chloride (C$_2$H$_5$Cl); Ethylene dichloride (C$_2$H$_4$Cl$_2$); Chloroform (CHCl$_3$).

Trichloroethylene is monitored by measuring urinary trichloracetic acid. Action level suggested: 60 μmol/mmol creatinine. No alcohol should be taken before sampling.

Methylene Chloride (Dichloromethane) RL 200 ppm.

Formerly regarded as one of the safest of the chlorinated hydrocarbons. However, recent work has shown that CO is one of the metabolites, and exposure to levels between 500 and 1000 ppm has resulted in up to 40% saturation with carboxyhaemoglobin. As the blood of smokers contains appreciable amounts of CO, monitoring is best done by measuring COHb at beginning and end of shift.

Carbon Tetrachloride (CCl₄) RL 10 ppm. Colourless liquid decomposed by heat into phosgene (COCl₂). Non-inflammable.
Uses: Has tended to be superseded by trichloroethane or perchlorethylene on account of toxicity.
 Formerly used in dry cleaning, as paint remover and as refrigerant.
 Still used in fire extinguishers.
Absorbed through skin. Narcotic and liver and kidney poison. May cause *toxic jaundice*, which is notifiable industrial disease.

Phosgene (COCl₂)

RL 0·1 ppm. Used in chemical industry as chlorinating agent. Produced when many chlorinated hydrocarbons are heated.
 Lung irritant with delayed action. Pulmonary oedema may follow absorption into alveoli with no sign of irritation of upper respiratory tract, because of low solubility in water. When this occurs, corticosteroids may be life-saving.

FLUORINE COMPOUNDS

Fluorine compounds occur naturally as fluorspar (calcium fluoride), cryolite (sodium aluminum fluoride) and fluorosilicates.

Hydrogen Fluoride (Hydrofluoric Acid)

TLV 3 ppm. Used for the cleaning, etching and frosting of glass, and the pickling of some metals; its most important industrial property is probably its solvent effect on glass.
 Inorganic fluorides are extensively used as fluxes. Can be monitored by urinary fluoride estimations — suggested limit 5 mg/l.
Toxic effects: Hydrogen fluoride is intensely corrosive to the skin, causing painful burns which are slow to heal. Inhalation of the vapour causes pulmonary oedema.
 Inunction with calcium gluconate gel is now the recommended first aid treatment for HF burns; having superseded injection, which is intensely painful.
 Long-term exposure to fluorides may cause osteosclerosis and mottling of dental enamel. If new bone formation encroaches on bone marrow anaemia may result. Fluorides can be absorbed through intact skin.
 Diagnosis is by X-ray. Fluoride excretion in urine is index of exposure.

Organic Fluorine Compounds

1. Fluorinated hydrocarbons are generally of low toxicity. TLVs of the commoner ones are 500–1000 ppm. Difluorodibromomethane is one of the most toxic (TLV 100 ppm).

They are used in fire extinguishers, as refrigerants, degreasers, and aerosol propellants. Many of them are decomposed by heat with formation of highly toxic breakdown products.

2. PTFE. Polymer of C_2F_4. Inert, but breakdown products when heated are toxic. (Over 300 °C.)

Polymer fume fever is an acute respiratory syndrome similar to metal fume fever — malaise, shivering, pyrexia and dyspnoea. Duration usually 24 hours. Smoking in contaminated atmosphere commonest cause.

3. Fluoracetic acid and derivatives (*see* Pesticides).

PHOSPHORUS

Organic Compounds

There is a wide and increasing range of organic phosphorus compounds, used as pesticides, as flame retardants and as plasticizers.

In general, they have two kinds of toxic effect — inhibition of cholinesterase, and delayed neurotoxicity (demyelination). For some compounds toxicity ratings have not been made, and Recommended Limits vary according to the compound.

Absorption occurs through the skin as well as by inhalation. Those in which neuronal damage predominates are the tri-aryl phosphates such as tri-ortho-cresyl phosphate (TOCP). Examples of pesticides which are, or may be, cholinesterase inhibitors are parathion, TEPP (tetraethylpyrophosphate) tri-ethyl phosphate, tris (2,3 dibromopropyl) thiosphosphate.

Early in 1977 disclosure of preliminary results of animal tests at the National Cancer Laboratory in USA revealed that tumours had been produced by the last of these, T23P, in experimental animals. Manufacture of it by American companies and their British subsidiaries thereupon ceased.

Acute poisoning: Headaches, giddiness, nausea and blurred vision are succeeded by vomiting and diarrhoea, sweating, muscular twitching, sphincter paralysis and pulmonary oedema. Coma and death may follow. Atropine should be given as soon as possible in 2-mg doses at 15-min intervals — intramuscularly or intravenously according to the degree of urgency. Respiration should of course be maintained meanwhile.

Subsequent treatment should be in a designated hospital — there are a number in each region — holding stocks of P25 (pralidoxine methane sulphonate) which is a specific antidote to some organophosphorus compounds.

Medical surveillance: Periodical estimations of red cell and plasma cholinesterase should be made, starting before first exposure to obtain base-line readings. The normal range of variation is wide; the lower limit is usually taken as 50 (expressed as a Cholinesterase Number derived from the pH), but in some individuals lower levels appear to be compatible with full health.

Red cell cholinesterase is the more significant reading, being specific for acetyl choline, but the non-specific enzyme in the plasma is more sensitive. A fall of 50% between consecutive readings requires removal from exposure for at least 3 weeks.

The effects of repeated absorption of small doses are cumulative.

Electromyography has been proposed as an alternative means of medical surveillance. It measures the electrical activity over the adductor pollicis when the ulnar nerve is stimulated at the wrist. Unfortunately responses are not specific to organophosphorus compounds, and they give no indication of CNS involvement.

(*See* Health and Safety Executive Memorandum MS 17: *Biological Monitoring of Workers Exposed to Organophosphorus Insecticides.*)

TOCP TLV 0.1 mg/m^3.

Effects on CNS: Attacks lower motor neurones, anterior horn cells, pyramidal tracts and spinocerebellar tracts.

Numbness and tingling of feet and hands followed by muscular pains, weakness, and ultimately lower motor neurone paralysis → foot and wrist-drop, muscular wasting.

Many survivors left with some permanent paralysis.

Yellow Phosphorus

TLV 0.1 mg/m^3. Ignites spontaneously when exposed to air. No longer used in industry, but is ingredient of incendiary bombs. May cause burns of skin and eyes.

Phosphine (PH₃)

TLV 0.3 ppm. Toxic gas smelling of garlic.

Evolved when slags contaminated with phosphorus are wet, in machining of spheroidal graphite iron and in treatment of ferro-silicon in presence of moisture; also by action of moisture on zinc phosphide used as rat poison.

Irritant to mucous membranes — may cause nose bleeds. Causes nausea and vomiting.

Irritant properties make chronic poisoning unlikely.

OTHER TOXIC CHEMICALS USED IN INDUSTRY

Ammonia (NH₃)

TLV 25 ppm. Colourless gas, freely soluble in water. Characteristic irritant odour.

Uses: Manufacture of fertilizers (sulphates and nitrates). Chemical and pharmaceutical industries. Refrigerant. Reducing agent in furnaces.

Acute poisoning: Caustic alkali. Inhalation — chemical burns of upper respiratory tract; cyanosis, dyspnoea, chemical pneumonitis. Irritation of skin and mucous membranes, especially conjunctivae.

Chronic poisoning: Does not occur.

Aniline and Bladder Carcinogens

Aniline 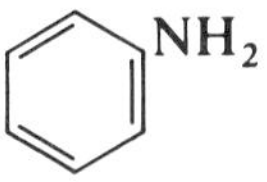   Made by reduction of nitrobenzene or amination of benzene, TLV 5 ppm, 10 mg/m^3.

Starting point for a large number of chemical processes.

Aniline and derivatives, when absorbed by man, cause cyanosis (anilism) by conversion of haemoglobin into methaemoglobin. Recovery is usually spontaneous 24 hours after exposure ceases.

Substances forming Methaemoglobin: Acetanilide; *o*- and *p*-Amino-phenol; Aniline; Dimethylaniline; Hydroxylamine; α- and β-Naphthylamine; *p*-Nitroaniline; Nitrobenzene; Nitroglycerine; Trinitrotoluene.

Known Bladder Carcinogens (variable latent period — usually over 10 years).

α-Naphthylamine

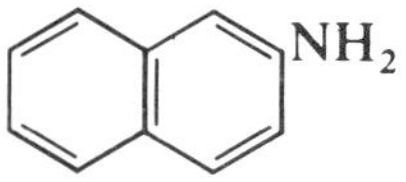

β-Naphthylamine

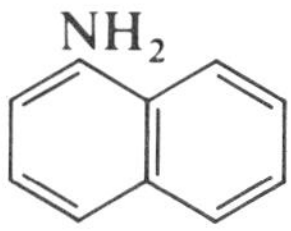

Benzidine

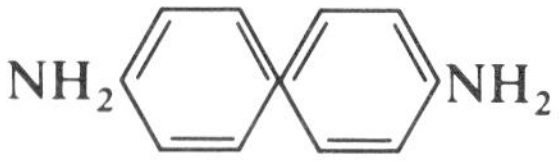

Dichlorbenzidine

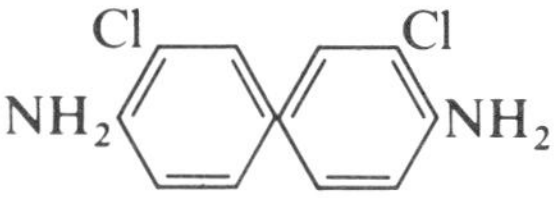

Orthotoluidine

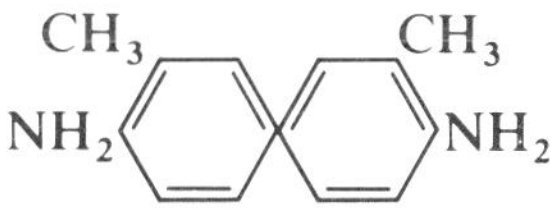

Dianisidine

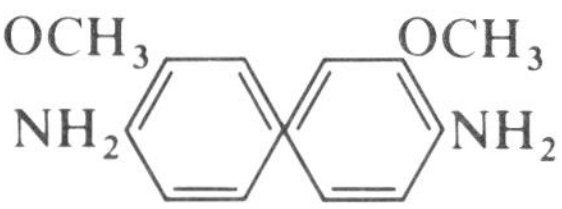

4-Aminodiphenyl

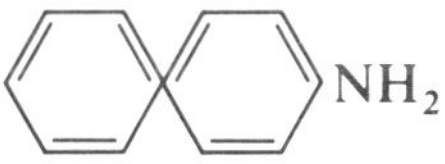

Carbon Monoxide (CO)

TLV 50 ppm, 55 mg/m³ in air. Colourless, odourless, non-irritant gas responsible for more than half of all industrial gassing fatalities.

Product of incomplete combustion of carbonaceous material.

Sources of exposure: Blast furnaces, coke ovens. Manufacture of water gas and producer gas. Space-heaters using solid fuel, gas or oil with inadequate ventilation. Exhaust from petrol engines. Manufacture of various organic compounds.

(Town gas, containing 5–20% of CO, was formerly a common source of exposure; but with the advent of natural gas, which contains no CO, traditional gas manufacture by carbonization of coal has virtually disappeared.)

Toxic effects: Formerly said to be purely due to anoxia. (CO combines with haemoglobin to form carboxyhaemoglobin, thus rendering it incapable of transporting oxygen to the tissues. Hb has affinity for CO 200–300 times that of oxygen and COHb breaks down less readily.) However, increasing evidence that at least some of the effects on the CNS are due to enzyme inhibition.

Symptoms depend on blood COHb levels.

Saturation of Carboxyhaemoglobin	Symptoms
0–10%	None.
10–20%	Tightness in head, dilatation of cutaneous blood vessels.
20–30%	Headache, throbbing at temples.
30–40%	Severe headache, nausea, vomiting, dizziness, blurring of vision, collapse.
40–50%	
50–60%	Syncope, rapid pulse, Cheyne–Stokes breathing, coma with convulsions.
Over 70%	Coma and death.

(The blood of smokers may contain 5–10% carboxyhaemoglobin and that of urban non-smokers 1–2%.)

Gassing with CO gives a pink tinge to the skin, due to the colour of COHb. Intellectual faculties, including judgement, are impaired, and drunkenness may be simulated.

Sequelae: Prolonged anoxia may cause permanent damage to:

CNS — mental retardation, psychosis, epilepsy, headaches, vertigo.

Cardiovascular system — angina, fibrillation, alteration to cardiac rhythm.

Kidneys — albuminuria and glycosuria.

(Sequelae of acute poisoning are not the same thing as *chronic CO poisoning.* Whether such a condition exists is a matter for controversy.)

Diagnosis of poisoning is confirmed by estimation of COHb. As this dissociates when exposed to air, blood samples must be kept in tubes from which air is excluded. Administration of oxygen helps the dissociation of COHb.

Not a notifiable industrial disease, but cases of industrial poisoning notifiable as Gassing Accidents. [Methylene chloride (dichloromethane) is metabolized to CO, so COHb estimation can also serve as a measure of its absorption.]

Cyanides. Hydrocyanic Acid, HCN; Cyanogen, CN; Sodium Cyanide, NaCN; Potassium Cyanide, KCN

Potassium and sodium cyanides are used in electroplating, steel hardening, and the extraction of gold and silver; they are also used as fumigants. Although they are highly toxic when ingested, the risk of industrial poisoning from inhalation is small. They can cause dermatitis.

They must, however, *never be allowed to mix with acid solutions*. This leads to the evolution of hydrogen cyanide, which is a highly toxic gas.

Hydrogen Cyanide TLV 10 ppm. Colourless gas smelling of bitter almonds. Inhibits enzyme required for transfer of oxygen from blood to tissues; hence asphyxia may occur even when blood is saturated with oxygen. Inhalation rapidly causes asphyxia and death.

Chronic poisoning is said to occur — symptoms of oxygen starvation, nausea, rapid pulse and headaches — all reversible. (When exposure is low, metabolized into thiocyanates, which are very much less toxic.)

Cyanogen is again a colourless gas smelling of bitter almonds, used as a fumigant and in certain manufacturing processes, and highly toxic.

Treatment of acute poisoning. The use of Kelocyanor Cyanide Kit is recommended by the Health and Safety Executive. This contains amyl nitrite capsules for crushing and immediate inhalation by the victim, and cobalt edetate for intravenous injection.

Caution. Cobalt edetate is itself quite toxic, and is only detoxified by the presence of circulating CN ions in the blood. It is therefore important to establish before giving it that the patient is in fact suffering from cyanide poisoning. False alarms are quite frequent, and when cyanide poisoning has not occurred, the injection may cause convulsions, rigors and collapse. It should *never* be given to a conscious patient. The notice supplied with the kit makes this point, saying injection should be given 'if the patient is unconscious or lapsing into unconsciousness' — but in the stress of an emergency, warning notices are not always read or absorbed.

Alternative intravenous injections are sodium nitrite (10 ml of a 3% solution) followed by 50 ml of 25% sodium thiosulphate; but in very many situations in industry it is unlikely that someone capable of giving an intravenous injection will be available in time to save a severely poisoned patient.

Apart from this, treatment is on general lines — artificial respiration, if required, supplemented by oxygen.

Ethylene Glycol Dinitrate

TLV 0·2 ppm.

$$CH_2-O-NO_2$$
$$|$$
$$CH_2-O-NO_2$$

Used as explosive, usually with nitroglycerine, than which it is much more volatile.

Absorbed through skin.

Exposure causes headache, flushing, tachycardia and fall in BP.

Sudden death from cardiac failure has been reported.

Glycol Ethers

These are used as solvents in very many manufacturing processes.

2-Methoxyethanol $CH_3-O-CH_2-CH_2-OH$ (methyl cellosolve, 2ME) and 2-ethoxyethanol $CH_3-CH_2-O-CH_2-CH_2-OH$ (cellosolve, 2EE) are used in the manufacture of lacquers, baking enamels and epoxy-resin coatings, and in printing inks, textile dyes and anti-icing fluids. 2EE is also used in varnish removers, thinners, cosmetics, pesticides and adhesives.

The acetates of both are also widely used in manufacturing industry.

Control limits: 2ME 25 ppm, 8-hour TWA; 2EE 200 ppm, 8-hour TWA.

They are toxic to the liver, kidney and CNS, and recent animal experiments suggest that they are teratogenic or lethal to the embryo, and may cause testicular atrophy and sterility in the male. It is safe to assume that structurally-related ethers such as 2-butoxyethanol, 2-phenoxyethanol and diethylene glycol dimethyl ether exert similar effects, pending the results of further animal tests. (US Department of Health and Human Services, Current Intelligence Bulletin 39, May 2, 1983.)

Ethylene Thiourea

Used as vulcanizing agent for neoprene synthetic rubber. Depressant of thyroid activity, and carcinogenic and teratogenic in rats. But none of these effects have so far been observed in rubber workers. It is, however, thought that the risk of teratogenicity is sufficient to justify exclusion of women of child-bearing age.

Formaldehyde (H.CHO)

TLV 2 ppm. Colourless gas, highly soluble in water, alcohol and ether. Pungent smell, detectable at less than 1 ppm.

Uses. Plastics production (urea formaldehyde, phenol formaldehyde, melamine formaldehyde resins).

Dyeing, tanning, photography.

Antiseptic and fungicide.

Toxicity relatively low, but irritant to mucous membranes at 2–3 ppm upwards. Acute poisoning by inhalation therefore unlikely, but ingestion of large amounts causes gastrointestinal symptoms, and ultimately convulsions and death.

Sensitizer, causing both skin reactions and asthma.

Has been suspected of carcinogenicity, because of mutagenic properties and results of animal experiments, but study of 605 men exposed for more than 5 years and followed for 20 years (Acheson et al., 1984) concluded no evidence for this — but proposed further studies.

A suggested method of monitoring exposure is by estimation of blood formic acid.

Hydrazine and Derivatives (NH₂NH₂)

TLV 0·1 ppm (hydrazine), 0·5 ppm (1,1, dimethylhydrazine), 5 ppm (phenyl).

Uses: Hydrazine and derivatives used in photography, metal processing and in manufacture of textile agents, pharmaceuticals and insecticides, and as rocket fuels. Isonicotinic acid hydrazide is used in the treatment of tuberculosis.

They are in general *absorbed through the skin* as well as the lungs, and are irritant to skin and mucous membranes, convulsants, hepatotoxic, and haemolysers; but the intensity of any of these effects varies somewhat with chemical composition.

Liver damage is the most important effect of chronic exposure.
Most are liquids at ordinary temperatures. BP (hydrazine) 113·5 °C.

Indulines

Blue purple dyes made from aniline. Induline is formed by a condensation reaction between aniline and sodium nitrite.

In May 1977 it was reported that 0·0–0·8% of 4-aminodiphenyl had been found in these dyes. This is a prohibited substance under the Carcinogenic Substances Regulations 1967, and has been shown to be carcinogenic in rats, mice, rabbits and dogs.

Manufacture of induline dyes has accordingly ceased, and warning letters advising periodical screening for carcinoma of the bladder by exfoliative cytology have been sent to customers of the manufacturers (Williams (Hounslow) Ltd) and to their own employees.

MOCA (MBOCA). Methylene-bis-orthochloroaniline

TLV 0·05 mg/m^3. Crystalline or granular solid at room temperature. MP 120 °C. Decomposes between 150 ° and 200 °C with evolution of toxic fumes. Automatic temperature control recommended in operation to shut down when temperature reaches 140 °C.

Uses: Manufacture of solid urethane, and of polyurethane foam with a hard outer skin.

In these processes, reacts with isocyanates (q.v.).

Toxic effects: Absorbed through skin. No evidence to date of carcinogenesis in man. However, it has caused haematuria in exposed workers, liver tumours in rats, and bladder tumours in dogs. Chemically it is related to a known potent carcinogen, 4,4, diamino-3,3 dimethyl-diphenylmethane.

Hence strict precautions should be taken to avoid skin contact and inhalation of vapour. Weighing and mixing, when done by hand, should be carried out in fume cupboards with extraction.

Biological monitoring: Urinary excretion can be estimated. There is no recognized 'safe' level of absorption, and it is the practice of DuPont, the original makers, to arrange immediate transfer if detectable amounts are found. This practice is recommended for UK also, and surveillance should continue until MOCA disappears from the urine. However, in UK the Health and Safety Executive has advised an interim upper limit of 10 μmol/creatinine, while also recommending that its use should be phased out as alternatives become available.

Phenol (C$_6$H$_5$OH) (Carbolic acid)

TLV 5 ppm, 19 mg/m^3. Colourless solid with characteristic odour. Produced by fractional distillation of coal tar.

Uses: Manufacture of plastics. Resins. Disinfectants. Dyes.

Hazard: Corrosive on skin and mucous membranes.

Acute poisoning: White staining of mouth, lips and skin. Abdominal pain. Burning sensation in mouth. Faintness, collapse and coma. No specific antidote.

Chronic poisoning: Rare. May include CNS and gastrointestinal disturbance. Urine dusky green, brown or black.

Trinitrotoluene

TLV 0·5 mg/m^3 in air. Yellow crystalline solid.

$$\underset{NO_2}{\overset{CH_3}{\underset{NO_2}{\bigcirc}NO_2}}$$

Used as high explosive. Not highly sensitive — requires detonation by more sensitive explosive.

Mainly absorbed through lungs, but some skin absorption may occur.

Stains skin and clothing yellow. Absorption causes cyanosis (anilism) through methaemoglobinaemia, toxic jaundice and toxic anaemia of aplastic type. A TNT gastritis with dyspepsia in the early morning is described.

Dermatitis may occur.

Webster Test on urine will detect presence of metabolites (aromatic amino compounds). (This is evidence of exposure, not intoxication.)

Pre-employment screening should exclude employees with history of liver disease or serious anaemia.

Toxic jaundice and toxic anaemia are notifiable industrial diseases.

Chemical Works Regulations (1922) apply to TNT, which is covered by the definition 'nitro- and amido-derivatives of benzene'.

Ozone (O$_3$)

TLV 0·1 ppm, 0·2 mg/m^3 in air. Gas with distinctive odour. Powerful oxidizing agent. Produced by high voltage discharges in air, e.g. welding with inert gases. Emitted from some forms of office duplicating machinery. Used in manufacture of paper and processing of oils and flour.

Effects of exposure: Irritant to mucous membranes at levels around TLV — cough, conjunctivitis.

Massive exposure causes pulmonary oedema — effect similar to nitrous fumes.

In experimental animals, has caused chromosomal changes and chronic pulmonary damage.

Odour is perceptible long before any irritant effects.

Long-term damage unlikely if no symptoms of irritation.

Silicones (Siloxanes)

Analogous to ketones — derived from hypothetical monomer $R_2Si=O$.

Wide range of polymers exists, using compounds with 1, 2, 3 or 4 functional oxygen atoms.

$$R_3Si-O-$$ Mono-functional (M)

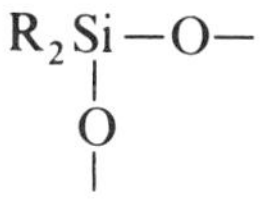

$$R_2Si-O-$$
$$\quad\quad |$$
$$\quad\quad O$$
$$\quad\quad |$$ Di-functional (D)

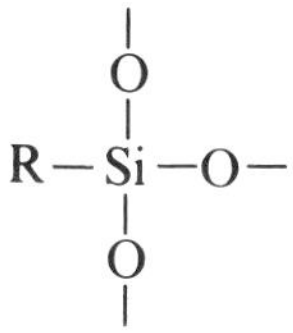

$$\quad\quad |$$
$$\quad\quad O$$
$$\quad\quad |$$
$$R-Si-O-$$ Tri-functional (T) 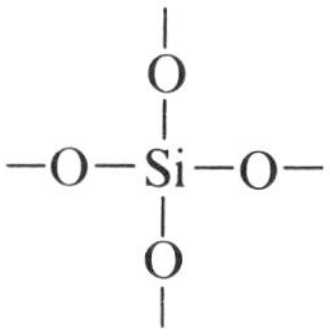
$$\quad\quad |$$
$$\quad\quad O$$
$$\quad\quad |$$

$$\quad\quad |$$
$$\quad\quad O$$
$$\quad\quad |$$
$$-O-Si-O-$$ Tetra-functional (Q)
$$\quad\quad |$$
$$\quad\quad O$$
$$\quad\quad |$$

These possess a wide variety of physical properties — hard, waxy, elastic, thermoplastic.

Siloxanes are most usually made by reacting silicon tetrachloride with alkyl or aryl magnesium chloride. Alkyl or aryl chlorosilanes are formed: these hydrolyse readily to form silanols, which polymerize by the conversion of Si–OH into Si–O–Si.

Methyl chlorosilanes and phenyl chlorosilanes are used for imparting a siloxane finish to paper and other materials. They appear to be non-toxic and non-irritant.

PLASTICS MANUFACTURE

Epoxy Resins

The reactive epoxy (ethoxylin) group is

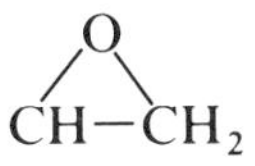

$$\overset{\displaystyle O}{\overset{\displaystyle /\backslash}{CH-CH_2}}$$

It reacts in the presence of caustic soda with polyhydroxy compounds to form an ether, and continuing polycondensation of this gives an epoxy resin.

$$\underset{H_2\ \ H\ \ H_2}{\overset{\displaystyle O}{\overset{\diagup\diagdown}{C}-C-C-Cl}} + HO-R-OH$$

Epichlorhydrin

↓ NaOH

$$\underset{H_2\ \ H\ \ H_2}{\overset{\displaystyle O}{\overset{\diagup\diagdown}{C}-C-C}}-O-R-O-\underset{H_2\ \ H\ \ H_2}{\overset{\displaystyle O}{C-\overset{\diagup\diagdown}{C}-C}} + NaCl + H_2O$$

Diglycidyl ether

The most commonly used polyhydroxy compound is 2,2 bis(*p*-hydroxy-phenyl) — propane(bisphenol A).

A large number of curing agents are used to produce thermosetting materials from the resins. These may react either with epoxy groups or with hydroxyl groups.

For hot curing, phthalic and maleic acid anhydrides.

For cold curing, amines, which may be secondary, tertiary or polyamines, or resins with free OH groups (phenoplasts and aminiplasts).

Uses: The cured resins have a wide range of uses — as glass fibre binding compounds, lacquer vehicles, glues, casting and textile treatment (crease resistance).

In general the resins and substances used in their manufacture are of low toxicity. Many of the resins and hardeners are both skin irritants and sensitizing agents, and all normal precautions against dermatitis are necessary. Cured resins are as a rule non-irritant and biologically inert, but may contain some unreacted material which may be released with heat or machining.

Isocyanates

Compounds containing $-N=C=O$ groups which react with polyols to form urethanes. Control Limit 0·02 ppm.

e.g.
$$R'-N=C=O$$
$$\underset{O}{\overset{N}{\underset{\|}{\overset{\|}{C}}}} \quad + \quad \underset{OH}{\overset{OH}{\underset{|}{\overset{|}{R''-OH}}}} \quad \longrightarrow \quad \overset{\displaystyle H}{\underset{O}{\underset{|}{-N}}\ \ \underset{|}{\overset{R'-N=C=O}{O-R''-O-}}}$$

Di-isocyanate   Polyhydroxy compound   Polyurethane

Toluene Di-isocyanate (TDI) (Desmodur T)
Highly volatile. BP 131 °C.

CH$_3$NCO

NCO

2 : 4 isomer

CH$_3$

OCH   NCO

2 : 6 isomer

Diphenyl-methane Di-isocyanate (MDI)
Non-volatile, BP 216 °C.

OCN⟨   ⟩—CH$_2$—⟨   ⟩NCO

Hexamethylene Di-isocyanate (HDI) (Desmodur H)
BP 132 °C. Highly volatile.

Naphthalene Di-isocyanate (NDI)
Non-volatile.
Uses:
1. In the foam industry. TDI usually used to make flexible foams, MDI rigid. Accelerator (freon) added. This produces CO_2 which is responsible for foam quality.
2. As lacquers, polishes and paints. Two-pack polyurethane paints contain isocyanates.
3. As adhesives.
4. In printing inks.

Toxic effects: Respiratory. Sensitization, producing asthmatic attacks. These may occur some hours after exposure ceases. Acute irritant effects on respiratory tract. Chronic alveolitis with interstitial fibrosis may occur, and has been recorded after acute over-exposure. *Skin:* Sensitization may occur. Less common than respiratory sensitization. *Eyes:* Irritant to conjunctiva.

Medical supervision: Pre-employment screening to eliminate those with history of allergies, pre-existing respiratory disease or impaired lung function.

Periodic tests of ventilatory capacity, e.g. Vitalograph.

Examination after more than 2 weeks' absence with respiratory disease.

The interpretation of lung function tests presents difficulties. There is no evidence that diminution of ventilatory capacity exceeding that due to ageing indicates susceptibility to sensitization.

Moreover, it cannot be assumed that sensitization does not occur at levels less than the Control Limit.

It has been established that in paint sprays and printing inks the airborne material is in the form of pre-polymers, i.e. isocyanates which have undergone the first stage of reaction with polyols; but these may carry with them residual unreacted isocyanates.

Polyester Resins

Saturated or unsaturated. Can be moulded by thermal or other treatment. Often reinforced with glass fibre. Formed by condensation reaction between alcohols and polybasic acids (e.g. terylene).

Alkyd Resins. Saturated dicarboxylic acids (chiefly phthalic acid anhydride) and polyalcohol (usually glycerol), e.g.

Phthalic acid anhydride   Glycerol   Fatty acid   Alkyd resin

Used in high-gloss paints, enamels, lacquers and varnishes.

Unsaturated Polyester Resins. Dicarboxylic acids (saturated or not) and dihydric alcohols with unsaturated dicarboxylic acids such as maleic acid anhydride.

Can be cross-linked with styrene   (Vinyl benzene $CH-CH_2$).

Cross-linking action with styrene usually slow; many polyesters supplied dissolved in styrene, e.g. methyl ethyl ketone peroxide, benzoyl peroxide, cumene hydroperoxide, dicumyl peroxide, lauroyl peroxide, acetyl peroxide, cyclohexanone peroxide.

Irritant to skin and mucous membranes especially eyes.

Organic peroxides used as catalysts.

Polyesters used in conjunction with glass fibre when rigid structure such as car body or boat hull required. Vinyl silane or methacrylate chromic chloride added to improve adhesion. Curing brought about by heat and pressure.

Health hazards: No evidence at present of lung hazard from cured resin — but it is a *skin irritant.*

So many possible starting points that no simple guide can be given to toxicology of polyester resin systems.

Styrene. Control Limit 100 ppm. Characteristic pungent smell. Defatting action may lead to dermatitis. Irritant to mucous membranes — eyes, nose, throat.

Inhalation → headache, fatigue, drowsiness, loss of balance, narcosis.

No firm evidence of long-term carcinogenic effect, but tumours have been reported in experimental animals.

Biological monitoring: Mandelic acid is a metabolite excreted in the urine and measurement of this is fairly accurate index of exposure. No alcohol should be taken in the hours before testing.

<5 SI Units — Low; 5–15 SI Units — Medium; > 15 SI Units — High (13 ≡ CL).

Acrylic Polymers

Monomer		*Polymer*
Acrylic acid	$H_2C=CH$ $\quad\overset{\displaystyle |}{C}\overset{\displaystyle O}{\diagup}$ $\quad\quad\diagdown OH$	→ Polyacrylic acid (ion-exchange medium)
Methylmethacrylate	$H_2C=C-CH_3$ $\quad\overset{\displaystyle |}{C}\overset{\displaystyle O}{\diagup}$ $\quad\quad\diagdown OCH_3$	→ Polymethylmethacrylate (Perspex)
Acrylonitrile (vinyl cyanide)	$H_2C=CH$ $\quad\overset{\displaystyle |}{CN}$	→ Polyacrylonitrile → Carbon fibres (Orlon)

Control Limit 24 ppm. Irritant to skin and mucous membranes. Sensitizer. Irritant to skin and mucous membranes. ?Hepatotoxic. ?Carcinogenic.

Note on Acrylonitrile. It has produced tumours in experimental animals, and DuPont et al. have reported that a study of workers on their polymerization plant had shown an excess incidence of cancer (of all sites). The survey is continuing.

Some of the acrylate compounds may be chlorinated, e.g. methyl or chloroacrylate methyl and β-dichloropropionate. These are highly irritant and may cause skin burns, blistering and keratitis.

Absorbed through skin.

Dimethylformamide $\left(\begin{array}{c} O \\ \| \\ HC-N \end{array} \diagup^{CH_3}_{\diagdown CH_3} \right.$ used as solvent for above.$\Big)$

TLV (skin) 10 ppm). Hepatotoxic; gastrointestinal disturbances.

Acrylamide H_2C-CH
$\quad\overset{\displaystyle |}{C}\overset{\displaystyle O}{\diagup}$
$\quad\quad\diagdown NH_2$

TLV (skin) 0·3 mg/m^3. *Absorbed through skin.*

Uses: Water-proofing sealant in tunnelling. Production of polymers in paper, textile, dyeing and photographic industries.

Irritant to skin and mucous membranes. Toxic to CNS — sympathetic overactivity, peripheral neuropathy, mid-brain disturbance.
Ethyl-2-cyanoacrylate

$$CH_2-\underset{\underset{CN}{|}}{C}-COOC_2H_5$$

Polymerizes in contact with moisture. Acts as powerful adhesive. Irritant to skin and mucous membranes. Sensitizer.

PESTICIDES AND HERBICIDES

The Agricultural (Poisonous Substances) Act 1952. Regulations under this Act require the provision of protective clothing for agricultural employees working with specific pesticides. Washing facilities and drinking water must also be provided.
Chemicals Specified under Regulations:

1. Di-nitro Compounds: Dinoseb (DNBP); DNOC; Medinoterb and salts.

Yellow dyes — colour evidence of exposure.

Metabolic stimulants — rapidly excreted. No permanent damage if poisoning not fatal.
Toxic effects: Fatigue, excessive sweating, thirst, insomnia, loss of weight.

Absorbed through skin.

Concentration in blood measurable. Removal from contact necessary if this exceeds 10 µg/ml.

No specific antidote.

2. Organochlorine Compounds: Endosulfan — Group includes DDT, aldrin, endrin, dieldrin, lindane, chlordane. (Aldrin and dieldrin are chlorinated naphthalenes: lindane is the gamma isomer of 1,2,3,4,5,6,-hexachlorocyclohexane.)
Absorbed through skin.
Toxic effects: On CNS. Muscular fibrillation, tremors, epileptiform convulsions.

Most compounds can be detected by direct estimation in blood.

3. Organophosphorus Compounds: Parathion, TEPP etc. (*See* pp. 167–8.)
Absorbed through skin.

4. Fluoracetic Acid Derivatives. Fluoroacetamide. Used as rat killer in ships' holds.

Absorbed through skin.
Toxic effects: Nausea, apprehension, muscular twitches, convulsions, cardiac irregularites.

Death may occur from cardiac and respiratory failure.

5. Organomercury Compounds. (*See* p. 158.)

6. Arsenic Compounds. (*See* p. 153.) Potassium arsenite. Sodium arsenite.

7. Organotin Compounds. Fentin acetate. Fentin hydroxide.

Toxic if ingested acting on CNS, but not readily absorbed through skin and human poisoning unknown.

8. Nicotine

Absorbed through skin

Toxic effects: Nausea, dizziness, vomiting, headache, tachycardia, sweating, followed by convulsions, respiratory depression, coma and death.

No specific antidote.

9. Paraquat and Diquat. These are bipyridylium compounds. Highly irritant to skin and mucous membranes.

Gastrointestinal symptoms, liver and kidney damage, late involvement of CNS. Ingestion of large amounts causes pulmonary oedema and haemorrhage. Smaller amounts, repeated, may cause pulmonary fibrosis and respiratory failure.

Latent period (2–3 days) may occur between swallowing and first symptom.

Detectable in urine. No specific antidote, but Fuller's Earth by mouth may delay absorption if given early. Treated by prolonged forced diuresis and symptomatically.

Cyanides, methyl bromide (q.v.) and ethylene dichloride are used as fumigants.

10. Carbamates. These are esters of carbamic acid whose toxicity to insects depends upon their action as cholinesterase inhibitors. This action is less powerful than that of organophosphorus insecticides, and is readily reversible; but periodic cholinesterase assays are advisable for monitoring the health of exposed workers, as for organophosphorus compounds.

Examples:

Carbaryl (Trade name Sevin)

Propoxur (Trade name Unden)

11. 2,4,5-T. This herbicide (2,4,5-trichlorophenol) is no longer used in some countries because of its supposed carcinogenic and teratogenic properties.

It is synthesized from 1,2,4,5-tetrachlorobenzene, and in the course of its manufacture the dioxin TCDD (2,3,7,8-tetrachlorodibenzo-*p*-dioxin) is formed as a by-product. TCDD is highly toxic to experimental animals, causing liver damage, cancers and damage to the embryo, and also chloracne and hyperkeratosis.

Chloracne has been observed in workers on plants making 2,4,5-T, but there have been a number of long-term studies which have failed to show any increase in cancers or congenital malformations in these people. Observations have been made in USA, Finland, New Zealand; on the other hand in Sweden it has been alleged that soft-tissue sarcoma is more prevalent in workers using the herbicide. The British Committee on Pesticides in 1982 concluded that it did not pose a safety hazard.

Chloracne is not life-threatening, and its occurrence is thought to be due to the presence of minute traces of TCDD. Further long-term mortality studies are clearly called for; but on the evidence at present available there does not seem to be a case for discontinuing the use of this material.

References

Approved Products for Farmers and Growers. Published in February each year by Ministry of Agriculture, Fisheries, and Food, Tolcarne Drive, Pinner, Middlesex HA5 2DT.
Encyclopedia of Occupational Health and Safety (1983) References to 2,4,5-T pp. 638, 746, 1034, 1616. Geneva, International Labour Office.
Poisonous Chemicals used on Farms and Gardens: Notes for the Guidance of Medical Practitioners. Department of Health and Social Security, Elephant & Castle, London SE1.

TARS

Tars are derived from the distillation of ligneous materials and coal; they contain a variety of aromatic hydrocarbons and their derivatives.

Coal Tar, and its heavy residue **Pitch**, contain the carcinogens 3,4-benzpyrene and 1,2,5,6-dibenzanthracene. Contact with the skin may cause erythema (tar smarts), keratotic patches (shagreen skin), tar keratoses, tar mollusca (warts) and tar epitheliomata. Cancer of the lung in gas workers is related to the inhalation of tar vapours from coal carbonization.

Asphalt (Bitumen) obtained by the distillation of petroleum is chemically and physically different from tar, containing bitumens and having a higher melting point. The vapour can cause irritation of the eyes and skin, acne-like lesions, mild keratoses and photosensitization. The high melting point prevents prolonged skin contact, skin cancer is not a hazard.

Bibliography

Browning, Ethel (1965) *Toxicity and Metabolism of Industrial Solvents.* Amsterdam, London & New York, Elsevier.
Browning, Ethel (1961) *Toxicity of Industrial Metals.* London, Butterworths.
CEMA's Notes of Guidance Health and Safety Executive, London.

Elsevier Monographs *The Halogenated Hydrocarbons of Industrial and Toxicological Importance* (1965). Von Oettingen.
  Industrial Toxicology and Dermatology in the Production and Processing of Plastics (1964). Malten & Zielhuis.
  Toxicity and Biochemistry of Aromatic Hydrocarbons (1960). Gerarde.
  Harmful Effects of Ionising Radiations (1959). Browning.
  Carcinogenic and Chronic Toxic Hazards of Aromatic Amines (1962). Scott.
  Toxic Aliphatic Fluorine Compounds (1959). Pattison.
Gosselin R., Hodge H. C., Smith and Gleason M. N. (1976) *Clinical Toxicology of Commercial Products*. 4th ed. Baltimore, Williams & Wilkins.
Encyclopedia of Occupational Health and Safety (1983) 3rd ed. Geneva, International Labour Office.
Patty, Frank A. (1963) *Industrial Hygiene and Toxicology*. Vol. II. Interscience Publishers.
Sax, N. Irving (1975) *Dangerous Properties of Industrial Materials*, 4th ed. New York, Van Nostrand Reinhold.
Schwartz, Tulipan and Birmingham. *Occupational Diseases of the Skin*. London, Kimpton.
Occupational Health and Safety. Geneva, International Labour Office.

HSE Publications

HSE Technical Data Notes (mostly superseded by later publications)
19 The ventilation of buildings: fresh air requirements
20 Anthrax
42 Probable asbestos dust concentrations at construction processes
52 Health hazards from sprayed asbestos coatings in buildings

Guidance Notes in the Environmental Hygiene Series
EH1   Cadmium — health and safety precautions
EH2   Chromium — health and safety precautions
EH4   Aniline — health and safety precautions
EH6   Chromic acid concentrations in air
EH7   Petroleum based adhesives in building operations
EH8   Arsenic — health and safety precautions
EH9   Spraying of highly flammable liquids
EH10 Asbestos — hygiene standards and measurements of airborne dust concentrations
EH11 Arsine — health and safety precautions
EH12 Stibine — health and safety precautions
EH13 Beryllium — health and safety precautions
EH14 Level of training for technicians making noise surveys
EH15 Threshold limit values for 1977
EH16 Isocyanates
EH17 Mercury
EH18 Precautionary policy for carcinogens
EH19 Antimony — health and safety precautions
EH20 Phosphine — health and safety precautions
EH21 Carbon dust — health and safety precautions
EH22 Ventilation of buildings — fresh air requirements
EH23 Anthrax — health hazards.
EH24 Dust and accidents in malt-houses
EH25 Cotton dust sampling
EH26 Occupational skin diseases — health and safety precautions
EH27 Acrylonitrile — personal protective equipment
EH28 Control of lead — air sampling techniques and strategies

EH29 Control of lead — outside workers
EH30 Control of lead — pottery and related industries
EH31 Control of exposure to polyvinyl chloride dust
EH32 Control of exposure to talc dust
EH33 Atmospheric pollution in car parks
EH34 Benzidine-based dyes — health and safety precautions
EH35
EH36
EH37
EH38 Ozone — health hazards and precautionary measures
EH40 Occupational exposure limits

Methods for the Detection of Toxic Substances in Air. Booklets describing simple and rapid means of measuring low concentrations in the atmosphere

 1 Hydrogen Sulphide
 2 Hydrogen Cyanide Vapour
 3 Sulphur Dioxide
 4 Benzene: Toluene and Xylene: Styrene
 5 Nitrous Fumes
 6 Carbon Disulphide Vapour
 7 Phosgene
11 Aniline Vapour
13 Mercury and Compounds of Mercury
17 Chromic Acid Mist
18 Ozone in the Presence of Nitrous Fumes
19 Hydrogen Fluroide and Other Inorganic Fluorides
20 Aromatic Isocyanates
21 Iron Oxide Fume
22 Copper Fume and Dust
23 Acetone
24 Isophorone
25 Zinc Oxide Fume
26 Cyclohexanone and Methylcyclohexanone

These and more recently published booklets can be obtained from the address below. In addition, HSE now publishes twice a year a Toxic Substances Bulletin, from the same address.

Further Information

Further advice on publications produced by the Executive is obtainable from any Area Office of the Health and Safety Executive, or from St. Hugh's House, Stanley Precinct, Bootle, Merseyside L20 3QY.

Chapter **15** *Toxicology III. Industrial Diseases*

NOTIFIABLE INDUSTRIAL DISEASES

Anthrax
Arsenic and arsine poisoning
Benzene poisoning
Beryllium poisoning
Cadmium poisoning
Cancer, occupational
Carbon disulphide poisoning
Chrome ulceration
Compressed air illness
Epitheliomatous ulceration
Lead poisoning
Manganese poisoning
Mercury poisoning
Phosphorus poisoning
Poisoning with nitro- and amido- derivatives of benzene (including trinitro-toluene, toxic jaundice, toxic anaemia)

CHEMICALS ABSORBED THROUGH SKIN

In general, these are fat-soluble, dissolving in alcohol, ether and other organic solvents, and insoluble in water.
Acrylamide
Acrylonitrile (vinyl cyanide)
Aniline and derivatives
Bromine
Carbon disulphide
Carbon tetrachloride and most other chlorinated hydrocarbons
Dimethyl formamide
Ethylene glycol trinitrate
Fluoracetic acid

Fluorides (inorganic)
Hydrazine and derivatives
Mercury (metal)
Methyl bromide (monobromomethane)
MOCA (MBOCA) (Methyl-bis-orthochloroaniline)
Nitro- and dinitro- derivatives of benzene
Nicotine
Organic lead (lead tetraethyl and tetramethyl)
Organic mercurials
Organochlorine compounds (DDT, aldrin, dieldrin, lindane, chlordane)
Organophosphorus compounds (parathion, malathion, TEPP)
Phenol and derivatives
Thallium and its salts
Trinitrotoluene
Turpentine

PRESCRIBED DISEASES

The list below includes the diseases covered by the Industrial Injuries scheme, with certain exceptions which are the subjects of special leaflets issued by the Department of Health and Social Security.

The exceptions, and the relevant leaflets, are:
Pneumoconiosis (leaflet NI.3; silicosis and asbestosis disease D.1 and byssinosis, disease D.2)
Occupational deafness, disease A.10, leaflet NI.207
Occupational asthma, disease D.7, leaflet NI.237.

Benefits Payable

There are two benefits payable under the industrial injuries scheme:

1. Disablement benefit — a payment which is dependent on the degree of disablement present either 90 days after the first day of incapacity for work or, alternatively, 90 days after the commencement of disablement due to the disease (whichever is the earlier). The size and duration of any assessment is determined by a medical board. Benefit is awarded by the insurance officer and is paid as either a lump sum or as a weekly pension. It can be paid concurrently with sickness or invalidity benefit.

2. Industrial death benefit — is payable to certain dependants if death is caused or materially accelerated by the prescribed disease.

From April 1983 special provision is made to pay sickness benefit to certain individuals, even though the normal contribution conditions are not satisfied, if they are employed earners who are incapable of working by reason of a prescribed disease.

In addition, for persons awarded disablement benefit, there are other allowances which may be paid, e.g. if the claimant cannot return to his own job or do work of an equivalent standard because of the disability arising from the relevant condition. Details of these allowances are set out in leaflets which can be obtained free of charge from local offices of the Department of Health and Social Security.

How Claims are Decided

Claims made under the industrial injuries scheme are decided by independent adjudicating authorities. There are two chains of adjudication, one which is non-medical and one which is medical. The non-medical chain of adjudication consists of an insurance officer, local tribunal and Social Security Commissioner. They deal with what are exclusively lay questions, e.g. did the claimant work in an occupation prescribed in relation to the disease claimed?

The adjudicating authorities on medical questions, i.e. diagnosis and recrudescence, are the insurance officer (who can give a decision on advice from a medical practitioner), the medical board (usually comprising two medical practitioners) and the medical appeal tribunal (which is made up of a legally qualified Chairman and two medical members of consultant status). To these authorities are reserved the strictly medical questions, but one question, that of causation, is decided by the insurance officer with appeals from his decision travelling along the lay adjudicating chain.

Pneumoconiosis, Byssinosis and Miscellaneous Diseases Benefit Scheme

This Scheme exists to provide benefits to claimants who develop certain diseases where the alleged causative employment took place prior to July 1948. The list of diseases covered by this Scheme is very restricted. They are pneumoconiosis; byssinosis; epitheliomatous cancer due to tar, pitch or other specified substances; disease of the skin due to X-rays, radium or other radioactive substances; nickel cancer; papilloma of the bladder; diffuse mesothelioma; and carcinoma of the nasal cavity or associated air sinuses.

Benefit is paid in respect of total or partial incapacity for work resulting wholly or partly from the disease or in respect of death caused or materially accelerated by such disease.

The list of prescribed diseases and the occupations for which they are prescribed follows.

Prescribed Disease or Injury	Nature of Occupation
A. Conditions due to physical agents	Any occupation involving:
1. Inflammation, ulceration or malignant disease of the skin or subcutaneous tissues or of the bones, or blood dyscrasia, or cataract, due to electromagnetic radiations (other than radiant heat), or to ionizing particles.	Exposure to electromagnetic radiations other than radiant heat, or to ionizing particles.

Prescribed Disease or Injury	Nature of Occupation
2. Heat cataract.	Frequent or prolonged exposure to rays from molten or red-hot material.
3. Dysbarism, including decompression sickness, barotrauma and osteonecrosis.	Subjection to compressed or rarefied air or other respirable gases or gaseous mixtures.
4. Cramp of the hand or forearm due to repetitive movements.	Prolonged periods of handwriting, typing or other repetitive movements of the fingers, hand or arm.
5. Subcutaneous cellulitis of the hand (Beat hand).	Manual labour causing severe or prolonged friction or pressure on the hand.
6. Bursitis or subcutaneous cellulitis arising at or about the knee due to severe or prolonged external friction or pressure at or about the knee (Beat knee).	Manual labour causing severe or prolonged external friction or pressure at or about the knee.
7. Bursitis or subcutaneous cellulitis arising at or about the elbow due to severe or prolonged external friction or pressure at or about the elbow (Beat elbow).	Manual labour causing severe or prolonged external friction or pressure at or about the elbow.
8. Traumatic inflammation of the tendons of the hand or forearm, or of the associated tendon sheaths.	Manual labour, or frequent or repeated movements of the hand or wrist.
9. Miner's nystagmus.	Work in or about a mine.
10. Occupational deafness.	(See Notes on Occupational Deafness).

B. Conditions due to biological agents

1. Anthrax.	Contact with animals infected with anthrax or the handling (including the loading and unloading or transport) of animal products or residues.
2. Glanders.	Contact with equine animals or their carcases.

Prescribed Disease or Injury	Nature of Occupation
3. Infection by Leptospira.	*a.* Work in places which are, or are liable to be, infested by rats, field mice or voles, or other small mammals; *b.* Work at dog kennels or the care or handling of dogs; *c.* Contact with bovine animals or their meat products or pigs or their meat products.
4. Ankylostomiasis.	Work in or about a mine.
5. Tuberculosis.	Contact with a source of tuberculous infection.
6. Extrinsic allergic alveolitis (including Farmer's Lung).	Exposure to moulds or fungal spores or heterologous proteins by reason of employment in: Any occupation involving: *a.* Agriculture, horticulture, forestry, cultivation of edible fungi or maltworking; or *b.* Loading or unloading or handling in storage mouldy vegetable matter or edible fungi; or *c.* Caring for or handling birds; or *d.* Handling bagasse.
7. Infection by organisms of the genus Brucella.	Contact with: *a.* Animals infected by brucella, or their carcases or parts thereof, or their untreated products; or with *b.* Laboratory specimens or vaccines of, or containing, brucella.
8. Viral hepatitis.	*a.* Close and frequent contact with human blood or human blood products; or *b.* Close and frequent contact with a source of viral hepatitis infection by reason of employment in the medical treatment or nursing of a

Prescribed Disease or Injury	Nature of Occupation
	person or persons suffering from viral hepatitis, or in a service ancillary to such treatment or nursing.
9. Infection by *Streptococcus suis*.	Contact with pigs infected by *Streptococcus suis*, or with the carcases, products or residues of pigs so infected.

C. Conditions due to chemical agents

1. Poisoning by lead or a compound of lead.	The use or handling of, or exposure to the fumes, dust or vapour of, lead or a compound of lead, or a substance containing lead.
2. Poisoning by manganese or a compound of manganese.	The use or handling of, or exposure to the fumes, dust or vapour of, manganese, or a substance containing manganese.
3. Poisoning by phosphorus or an inorganic compound of phosphorus or poisoning due to the anticholinesterase or pseudo-anticholinesterase action of organic phosphorus compounds.	The use or handling of, or exposure to the fumes, dust or vapour of, phosphorus or a compound of phosphorus or a substance containing phosphorus.
4. Poisoning by arsenic or a compound of arsenic.	The use or handling of, or exposure to the fumes, dust or vapour of, arsenic or a compound of arsenic, or a substance containing arsenic.
5. Poisoning by mercury or a compound of mercury.	The use or handling of, or exposure to the fumes, dust or vapour of, mercury or a compound of mercury, or a substance containing mercury.
6. Poisoning by carbon bisulphide.	The use or handling of, or exposure to the fumes or vapour of, carbon bisulphide or a compound of carbon bisulphide, or a substance containing carbon bisulphide.

Prescribed Disease or Injury	Nature of Occupation
7. Poisoning by benzene or a homologue.	The use or handling of, or exposure to the fumes of, or vapour containing benzene or any of its homologues.
8. Poisoning by a nitro- or amino- or chloro-derivative of benzene or of a homologue of benzene, or poisoning by nitrochlorbenzene.	The use or handling of, or exposure to the fumes of, or vapour containing a nitro- or amino- or chloro-derivative of benzene or nitrochlorbenzene.
9. Poisoning by dinitrophenol or a homologue or by substituted dinitrophenols or by the salts of such substances.	The use or handling of, or exposure the fumes of, or vapour containing, dinitrophenol or a homologue or substituted dinitrophenols or the salts of such substances.
10. Poisoning by tetrachloroethane.	The use or handling of, or exposure to the fumes of, or vapour containing tetrachloroethane.
11. Poisoning by diethylene dioxide (dioxan).	The use or handling of, or exposure to the fumes of, or vapour containing diethylene dioxide (dioxan).
12. Poisoning by methyl bromide.	The use or handling of, or exposure to the fumes of, or vapour containing, methyl bromide.
13. Poisoning by chlorinated naphthalene.	The use or handling of, or exposure to the fumes of, or dust or vapour containing chlorinated naphthalene.
14. Poisoning by nickel carbonyl.	Exposure to nickel carbonyl gas.
15. Poisoning by oxides of nitrogen.	Exposure to oxides of nitrogen.
16. Poisoning by gonioma kamassi (African boxwood).	The manipulation of gonioma kamassi or any process in or incidental to the manufacture of articles therefrom.
17. Poisoning by beryllium or a compound of beryllium.	The use or handling of, or exposure to the fumes, dust or vapour of, beryllium, or a substance containing beryllium.

Prescribed Disease or Injury	Nature of Occupation
18. Poisoning by cadmium.	Exposure to cadmium dust or fumes.
19. Poisoning by acrylamide monomer.	The use or handling of, or exposure to, acrylamide monomer.
20. Dystrophy of the cornea (including ulceration of the corneal surface) of the eye.	*a.* The use or handling of, or exposure to, arsenic, tar, pitch, bitumen, mineral oil (including paraffin), soot or any compound, product or residue of any of these substances except quinone or hydroquinone; *b.* Exposure to quinone or hydroquinone during their manufacture.
21. *a.* Localized new growth of the skin, papillomatous or keratotic. *b.* Squamous-celled carcinoma of the skin.	The use or handling of, or exposure to, arsenic, tar, pitch, bitumen, mineral oil (including paraffin), soot or any compound, product or residue of these substances except quinone or hydroquinone.
22. *a.* Carcinoma of the mucous membrane of the nose or associated air sinuses. *b.* Primary carcinoma of a bronchus or of a lung.	Work in a factory where nickel is produced by decomposition of a gaseous nickel compound which necessitates working in or about a building or buildings where that process or any other industrial process ancillary or incidental therto is carried on.
23. Primary neoplasm (including papilloma, carcinoma-in-situ and invasive carcinoma) of the epithelial lining of the urinary tract (renal pelvis, ureter, bladder and urethra).	*a.* Work in a building in which any of the following substances is produced for commercial purposes: (i) alpha-naphthylamine, beta-naphthylamine or methylene-bis-orthochloroaniline; (ii) diphenyl substituted by at least one nitro or primary amino group or by at least one nitro and primary amino group (including benzidine);

Prescribed Disease or Injury	Nature of Occupation
	(iii) any of the substances mentioned in sub-paragraph (ii) above if further ring substituted by halogeno, methyl or methoxy groups, but not by other groups;
	(iv) the salts of any of the substances mentioned in sub-paragraph (i) to (iii) above;
	(v) Auramine or magenta;
	b. The use or handling of any of the substances mentioned in paragraph *a*, except auramine and magenta (sub-paragraph v), or work in a process in which any such substance is used or handled or is liberated;
	c. The maintenance or cleaning of any plant or machinery used in any such process as is mentioned in paragraph *b* or the cleaning of clothing used in any such building as is mentioned in paragraph *a* if such clothing is cleaned within the works of which the building forms a part or in a laundry maintained and used solely in connection with such works.
24. *a*. Angiosarcoma of the liver. *b*. Osteolysis of the terminal phalanges of the fingers. *c*. Non-cirrhotic portal fibrosis.	*a*. Work in or about machinery or apparatus used for the polymerization of vinyl chloride monomer, a process which, for the purposes of this provision, comprises all operation up to and including the drying of the slurry produced by the polymerization and the packaging of the dried product; or *b*. Work in a building or structure in which any part of that process takes place.

Prescribed Disease or Injury	Nature of Occupation
25. Occupational vitiligo.	The use or handling of, or exposure to, para-tertiary-butylphenol, para-tertiary-butylcatechol, para-amyl-phenol, hydroquinone or the monobenzyl or monobutyl ether of hydroquinone.

D. Miscellaneous conditions not included elsewhere in this Schedule

Prescribed Disease or Injury	Nature of Occupation
1. Pneumoconiosis.	Employed earner's employment of a type specified in regulation 2(b) and in Part II of this Schedule.
2. Byssinosis.	Work in any room in a factory where any process up to and including the weaving of cotton or flax is performed.
3. Diffuse mesothelioma (primary neoplasm of the mesothelium of the pleura or of the pericardium or of the peritoneum).	*a.* The working or handling of asbestos or any admixture of asbestos. *b.* The manufacture or repair of asbestos textiles or other articles containing or composed of asbestos. *c.* The cleaning of any machinery or plant used in any of the foregoing operations and of any chambers, fixtures and appliances for the collection of asbestos dust. *d.* Substantial exposure to the dust arising from any of the foregoing operations.
4. Inflammation or ulceration of the mucous membrane of the upper respiratory passages or mouth produced by dust, liquid or vapour.	Exposure to dust, liquid or vapour.
5. Non-infective dermatitis of external origin (including chrome ulceration of the skin but excluding dermatitis due to ionizing or electromagnetic radiations other than radiant heat).	Exposure to dust, liquid or vapour or any other external agent capable of irritating the skin (including friction or heat but excluding ionizing particles or electromagnetic radiations other than radiant heat).

Prescribed Disease or Injury	Nature of Occupation
6. Carcinoma of the nasal cavity or associated air sinuses (nasal carcinoma).	*a.* Attendance for work in or about a building where wooden goods are manufactured or repaired; or
	b. Attendance for work in a building used for the manufacture of footwear or components of footwear made wholly or partly of leather or fibre board; or
	c. Attendance for work at a place used wholly or mainly for the repair of footwear made wholly or partly of leather or fibre board.
7. Asthma which is due to exposure to any of the following agents:	Exposure to any of the agents set out in column 1 of this paragraph.
a. Isocyanates.	
b. Platinum salts.	
c. Fumes or dusts arising from the manufacture, transport or use of hardening agents (including epoxy resin curing agents) based on phthalic anhydride, tetrachlorophthalic anhydride, trimellitic anhydride or triethylene-tetramine.	
d. Fumes arising from the use of rosin as a soldering flux.	
e. Proteolytic enzymes.	
f. Animals or insects used for the purposes of research or education or in laboratories.	
g. Dusts arising from the sowing, cultivation, harvesting, drying, handling, milling, transport or storage of barley, oats, rye, wheat or maize, or the handling, milling, transport or storage of meal or flour made therefrom (occupational asthma).	

SUMMARY OF TOXIC EFFECTS

This list is not complete; it is intended as an *aide-mémoire* for the student, who can make his own additions. Most toxins involve the liver (metabolism) and the kidney (excretion) but this summary notes the main toxic effects.

Toxic Jaundice. TNT; dinitrophenol; dinitro-orthocresol; dinitrobenzene; carbon tetrachloride; tetrachloroethane; chlorinated naphthalenes; dioxan; stibine; ethylene chlorhydrin; phosphorus; hydrazine.

Toxic Nephritis. Cadmium; mercury; arsine; lead; thallium; paraquat.

Haemolytic Anaemia. Arsine; stibine; tin tetrahydride; aniline; phenylhydrazine; toluene diamine; Weil's disease.

Anaemias and Blood Dyscrasias. Lead; benzene; TNT; DNOC, DNB; arsenic; ionizing radiations.

Peripheral Nervous System. Parathion; lead; arsenic; thallium; dinitrophenol; triorthocresylphosphate; acrylonitrile.

Central. Lead; manganese; mercury; aniline; carbon disulphide; benzene; methyl alcohol; methyl bromide; methyl chloride; glycols; acrylonitrile.

Toxic Psychosis. Mercury; lead; carbon disulphide; DNOC; endrin.

Nasal Septum Ulceration. Mercury fulminate; chromic acid and chromates; soda ash; cement; arsenic; organic mercurials.

Occupational Asthma. Cigarette cutters; cotton workers; printers (gum acacia); flax; grain; farmers' lung; wood dust; isocyanates; vanadium pentoxide; carbaryl (Sevin); formaldehyde; resins, especially colophony and epoxy.

Cataract. DNOC; naphthalene; hydrogen sulphide; thallium; mercury (mercurialentis).

INDUSTRIAL LUNG DISEASES

The lungs are the most important portal of entry for most industrial poisons. Those which are absorbed cause systemic effects; the name pneumoconiosis is given to those dust diseases affecting the respiratory tract. The most serious of these are associated with fibrosis.

Dust particles above 5 μm in diameter do not penetrate into alveoli.

Silicosis is due to inhalation of silica (silicon dioxide).

Nodular fibrosis beginning around aggregations of lymphoid tissue.

Coal workers' pneumoconiosis is modified form due to mixed dust in coal mining.

Other processes with hazard include: Fettling in foundries. Sand blasting. Making of abrasive soaps and scouring powders. Mining of gold and haematite. Grinding of metals. Pottery manufacture.

Symptoms are increasing dyspnoea, non-productive cough and pain in chest, progressing to compensatory emphysema and cor pulmonale. Bronchitis frequently occurs in association.

Diagnosis by X-ray (q.v.).

Asbestosis. Silicates of magnesium, sometimes containing iron.

Main varieties: Chrysotile, amosite, anthophyllite, crocidolite (blue asbestos). Total annual imports now 200 000 tons.

First reported industrial use in 1890.

1900 First reported case of asbestosis.

1924 Second reported case of asbestosis.

1928–9 Survey of asbestos workers by Merewether and Price. Fibrosis found in one-third of those examined.

1932 Asbestos Regulations (requiring in general terms adequate ventilation of workrooms).

1950–60 Measurement techniques for airborne dust developed.

1960 American standard set at 177 particles/cc.

1964 Association with mesothelioma found (mainly with crocidolite exposure).

1969 New Asbestos Regulations (setting permissible limit at 2 fibres/cc in air).

1970 Import of crocidolite into UK ceases.

1983 New control limits adopted:

For dust consisting of or containing any crocidolite (blue asbestos):

0·2 fibre/ml when measured as time-weighted average over any 4-hour period.

For dust consisting of or containing any amosite (brown asbestos) but not crocidolite:

0·5 fibre/ml when measured as time-weighted average over any 4-hour period.

For dust consisting of or containing other types of asbestos (e.g. chrysotile — white asbestos) but nor crocidolite or amosite:

1 fibre/ml when measured as time-weighted average over any 4-hour period.

In 1983 also, an Approved Code of Practice and Guidance Note for work covered by the Asbestos Regulations of 1969 was issued by the Health and Safety Executive. It stresses that the figures quoted do not represent 'safe' levels and there is a statutory duty to reduce exposure to lower levels if reasonably practicable.

Effects of exposure.

1. Asbestos bodies in sputum. (Sign of *exposure*, not disease.)

2. Pleural thickening and plaques. (Appearance on X-ray indicates *exposure*, not disease.)

3. Asbestosis. Progressive fibrosis of insidious onset causing dyspnoea and cough. May first appear long after exposure ceases.

4. Lung and bronchial cancer. Risk higher in asbestosis than in general population. Enhanced by cigarette smoking.

5. Mesothelioma. Mainly associated with crocidolite but ?possibly with other forms of asbestos. Exposure may have been brief, and not necessarily occupational. Long latent period. 65% of cases estimated as due to occupational exposure.

There appears to be no constant association between asbestosis and mesothelioma but they may coexist.

In a report to the Health and Safety Commission in 1983, Acheson and Gardner* concluded that no new evidence had arisen since 1979 to alter substantially the conclusions which they then reached in a report to the Advisory Committee† on asbestos; but they would be modified in the following respects:

'Amosite imports have effectively ceased, and chrysotile is at present for practical purposes the only type of raw asbestos imported into the UK.

'The evidence that asbestos fibre causes alimentary tract cancer in man is less convincing than in 1979.

'The case that amosite is more dangerous than chrysotile has been strengthened in respect of both peritoneal and pleural mesothelioma. We recommend that formal prohibition of the manufacture and importation of new products made of amosite and crocidolite should be considered.'

They concluded also that there was a linear relationship between mortality from lung cancer and exposure to asbestos, and that peritoneal mesothelioma had never, and pleural mesothelioma rarely, occurred in human beings after exposure to white asbestos alone. They advised further improvements in asbestos control and the gradual curtailment of the use of all types of asbestos, and further epidemiological studies on the asbestos cement industry, where chrysotile only has been used.

Benefit for asbestosis. Payable under Industrial Injuries Scheme on assessment made by Pneumoconiosis Medical Panel.

Asbestosis is invariably due to occupational exposure, mainly in asbestos factories and insulation industry. New cases at present total about 160 annually. Insulation industry no longer uses asbestos on new work, but workers may encounter it in stripping old lagging and in demolition work. Sprayed asbestos is not longer used.

Mesothelioma cases number at present about 200 per year.

Crocidolite hazard still exists in demolition work. Every contractor must obtain clearance from Factory Inspector before beginning demolition of buildings or plant containing crocidolite, and stringent precautions must now be taken to protect workers and in disposal of waste.

It will be 10–20 years before the application of stricter environmental standards will be reflected by a drop in the incidence of both asbestosis and mesothelioma, as is hoped.

Byssinosis. Asthma and chronic bronchitis occurring in card room workers in cotton spinning mills. Characteristic feature is 'Monday tightness' and cough — worse on Monday after week-end break.

Allergic response to some ingredient of cotton plant most of which is removed in earliest stages of preparation of cotton fibres for spinning.

* Acheson E. D. and Gardner M. J. (1983) The Control Limit for asbestos. Health and Safety Commission. London, HMSO.
† Health and Safety Commission. Asbestos: Vol. 2: Final Report of the Advisory Committee, 1979.

No characteristic X-ray changes. Diagnosis rests mainly on questionnaire. Compensable only in workers with 10 years or more in card rooms or blowing rooms (but does occur in later stages of spinning process).

Bagassosis. Similar to byssinosis. Due to inhalation of dust from fibres left after extraction of sugar from cane.

Farmer's Lung. Allergic phenomenon due to moulds and fungi (mainly Aspergillus) found in damp hay and straw.

Berylliosis. Granulomatosis affecting lungs and other organs. (*See* beryllium.)

Tin, Iron and Barium cause X-ray changes without fibrosis or impairment of lung function.

Talc (Hydrated Magnesium Silicate) can cause pulmonary fibrosis with emphysema.

X-RAY DIAGNOSIS OF PNEUMOCONIOSIS

The International Classification of Radiographs of Pneumoconiosis (1971) uses standard films for limits of normality, and uses the following system:
p   rounded opacities up to 1·5 mm diameter.
q(m)   rounded opacities between 1·5 and 3 mm diameter.
v(n)   rounded opacities between 3 mm and 1 cm diameter.
s   fine irregular or linear opacities.
t   medium irregular opacities.
u   coarse irregular opacities.
Profusion of Small Opacities. Defined by standard films.
Category 0 small opacities absent.
Category 1 small opacities present, but few in number.
Category 2 small opacities numerous. Lung markings partly obscured.
Category 3 small opacities very numerous. Lung markings totally obscured.
Intermediate categories recognized. If category above or below that used is seriously considered as alternative, this is recorded second, thus: 1/1, 2/3.
Hence full spectrum of categories is: 0,0/0, 1/0, 1/1, 1/2, 2/1, 2/2, 2/3, 3/2, 3/3, 3/4.
Zones in which opacities are seen are recorded — upper, mid and lower zones in each lung defined by horizontal lines at one-third and two-thirds of vertical distance between apex of lung and dome of diaphragm.
Large opacities are recorded according to size.
Extent, width and site of pleural thickening recorded, and obliteration of costophrenic angle and pleural calcification.
Diaphragmatic and cardiac outlines recorded
See also Guidelines for the Use of ILO International Classification of Radiographs

of Pneumoconioses. Revised Edition, 1980. ILO Occupational Health and Safety Series No. 22. Geneva.

DERMATITIS

The terms 'dermatitis' and 'eczema' are synonymous; but to the layman dermatitis is usually thought to imply a skin condition due to occupation.

Characteristic lesions are erythema, accompanied by irritation, vesiculation, weeping following the rupture of vesicles, crusting, desquamation, and lichenification. Any or all of these may coexist at any given time.

Occupational causes of dermatitis fall into two groups:

Primary Irritants. These are substances which will irritate and damage any skin if contact is sufficiently heavy and prolonged. They include strong acids and alkalis and fat solvents, and also physical agents such as heat, friction and radiation. Lesions are confined to exposed areas of skin, and clear up rapidly after removal from contact with the irritant.

Sensitizers. Sensitization may occur after a long period of exposure which has produced no ill effects. It is an allergic response, personal to the individual, and sensitizing agents include animal, vegetable and mineral products; but on the whole they tend to be substances with complex rather than simple molecular structure. Some primary irritants may also act as sensitizers.

Lesions tend to occur initially on exposed areas of skin, but may quickly spread to involve other areas of the body. There may be oedema of the orbits. The appearances do not differ at all from those of a non-occupational or constitutional eczema; for this reason differential diagnosis does not depend on any objective criteria, but rests much more on careful history taking and knowledge of the existence of cases in other workers similarly exposed. Often an opinion on occupational causation rests purely on a balance of probabilities — it is impossible to be dogmatic, and usually unwise to try.

Sensitization is usually long-lasting, if not permanent, and more than one recurrence on return to the same work after recovery will as a rule mean that the worker should be advised to change his or her job.

Occupational dermatitis, contrary to popular lay belief, is not contagious, and it may be important to reassure patients on this point.

However, epidermophytosis of the feet (athlete's foot) can be a contagious occupational disease, spread by walking in bare feet in baths and showers. It may trigger off a constitutional eczema, or a reaction to an occupational irritant. Diagnosis of a recent eczematous eruption should therefore always include inspection of the interdigital clefts of the toes.

Prevention follows standard principles:

1. Substitution of the irritant substance, where practicable.
2. Enclosure of the process.
3. Personal protection, e.g. gloves, barrier creams. Barrier creams are of limited value; they are rarely thoroughly and properly applied to those areas needing protection — the dorsum of the hands and the interdigital clefts; and they

quickly rub off, and require re-application at frequent intervals, which in practice is seldom done. They have, however, a place as part of a general policy of prevention.

4. Selection of workers. There is no reliable way of predicting in advance which workers are liable to develop dermatitis; but if the job entails contact with a known sensitizer, it is wise to exclude people with a history of atopy in any form. Patch tests have no place in pre-employment selection — a negative result gives no guarantees for the future.

Treatment. This is empirical rather than specific. Essential factors are:

Removal from contact with the irritant.

Application of an antipruritic — corticosteroids are now most commonly used — to break the vicious circle of itch/scratch/more itch.

Covering of the affected areas to minimize external irritation, prolong the efficacy of the topical application, and prevent scratching.

Probing to determine and discuss causes of anxiety, stress and insecurity, occupational or personal. The patient's mental attitude is an important factor in the prognosis and this aspect with reassurance when justified is as essential as local treatment.

ANTHRAX

Bacillus anthracis causes in cattle, sheep, horses, pigs and goats an illness which is usually fatal (gastroenteritis followed by septicaemia).

Man may be infected by handling infected material. Disease rare among animals in Britain; human infection usually contracted from imported material — hides, skins, hair, wool, hoof and horn, bone meal. Now rare (<10 cases annually).

Commonest form is a skin lesion known as malignant pustule; but gastrointestinal and pulmonary infections also occur in man.

Malignant pustule usually in exposed area — forearm, neck or face. Papule progressing to vesicle with surrounding oedema, then central necrosis with formation of black slough.

Pulmonary form now very rare — in past always fatal.

Disease usually responds to antibiotics (mainly penicillin). Sclavo's serum used for toxaemia.

Satisfactory active immunization possible by vaccination.

Numerous Orders and Regulations for control apply in specific industries.

Anthrax Prevention Order 1971 makes disinfection of certain classes of imported hair and wool obligatory.

Notifiable and prescribed industrial disease.

BRUCELLOSIS

May be contracted by drinking milk infected with *Brucella abortus* and by veterinary workers with infected cattle.

Protracted illness characterized by malaise, intermittent pyrexia, and often causing serious depression.

CATTLE RINGWORM

Fungal infection of skin acquired from cattle by dairymen.

ERYSIPELAS

Rosenbach's erysipeloid is a cutaneous infection affecting fish handlers, caused by the organism producing swine erysipelas. Trauma a factor — possibly also allergy.
   A more serious septicaemic form, with endocarditis, may occur.

FARMER'S LUNG

Allergic pneumonitis, formerly thought to be a mycosis, due to inhalation of Aspergillus spores from mouldy hay, but now believed to be allergic response to spores of *Micropolyspora foeni*. Acute illness may be short, with severe dyspnoea on exertion: subacute may be seen after repeated exposure. Chronic disease with fibrosis and emphysema rarely occurs. Prescribed industrial disease in farm workers (but self-employed farmers not eligible for industrial injury benefit).

GLANDERS

Acquired from horses by grooms and others in close contact with them. Pulmonary and cutaneous forms. Amputation often necessary in past.
   Historical interest only — disease now extinct in horses and man.

WARTS

Virus warts are relatively common in some occupations, notably fish filleters and those using glue.

WEIL'S DISEASE (LEPTOSPIROSIS)

Leptospirosis is thought to be the most widespread zoonosis in the world. The natural reservoir for many leptospires is wild animals, particularly the rodent family. Domestic animals, such as dogs, or farm livestock may also become infected, either directly with leptospiral serogroups specific for their species, e.g. Canicola in dogs and *Hebdomadis serovar hardjo* in cattle; or indirectly by contact with contaminated urine from another host, e.g. dogs with Icterohaemorrhagiae. Man is an accidental host. The host animal is often asymptomatic but will carry leptospira in high numbers in the kidneys, excreting them in the urine to rivers, canals and animal feedstuffs on farms. Leptospires enter the body through cuts and abrasions of the skin or by contact with mucous membrane of the nose, mouth or eyes.

Table 16.1. Human leptospira cases in the British Isles, 1983

Icterohaemorrhagiae	39 (32%)
Hebdomadis (hardjo)	55 (46%)
Canicola	8 (7%)
Others/not determined	18 (15%)
Total	120

Sewer workers are now less commonly infected with Weil's disease, probably as a result of modern pest control measures, the use of protective clothing and the presence in waste waters of detergents which rapidly destroy leptospires. The majority of cases of Icterohaemorrhagiae and Hebdomadis (hardjo) now occur in the farming industry. (*See also* p. 93.)

Table 16.2. Serogroup *Hebdomadis serovar hardjo* cases in 1983

Occupation	Number
Farming	
Arable	—
Cowmen	25
Dairy farmers	17
Sheep farmers	1
Beef farmers	1
Others	
Meat inspectors	1
Butchers	1
Veterinarians	2
Miscellaneous	7
Total	55

(From 'Update on Leptospirosis', Public Health Laboratory Service. *British Medical Journal*, 1985, **290**, 1502.)

STREPTOCOCCUS SUIS

Porcine streptococci can cause meningitis and septicaemia in man. Cases have been reported in the Netherlands and Britain in pig breeders, slaughterhouse workers and other people who may have handled meat from infected pigs.

DOGGER BANK ITCH

Eczematous dermatitis due to sensitization to the sea-chervil, *Alyconidium hirsutum*. This is a marine animal growing in colonies which may be drawn in with the nets. Hands primarily affected; eruption may spread to face and other parts.

NEWCASTLE DISEASE

Disease of fowls which can be transmitted to humans. Features are unilateral conjunctivitis, tenderness and enlargement of pre-auricular gland on same side, with malaise and headache but no pyrexia. Complete recovery usual within 1–2 weeks.

PIGEON FANCIER'S LUNG

Condition similar to farmer's lung caused by antigens in the droppings of pigeons and other birds (extrinsic allergic alveolitis). Specific antibodies are found in the serum, and symptoms thought to be result of precipitin mediated hypersentivity reaction.

HUMIDIFIER FEVER

Fever and malaise with influenza-like symptoms thought to be an extrinsic allergic alveolitis caused by spores of fungi growing in humidifiers and water cooling systems. May hitherto have been unrecognized, symptoms being attributed to infection.

Legionnaires' Disease, due to a specific micro-organism, is spread in a similar way.

Sick Building Syndrome. This label has been used to describe non-specific symptoms arising in staff who work in buildings which are artificially ventilated. Air is recirculated and filtered with an adjustment for humidity and temperature. Various instances have been reported of staff complaining of rhinitis, headaches, lethargy and sore eyes. These symptoms can occur even if investigations exclude humidifier fever or legionnella.

Bibliography

Finnegan M., Pickering C. A. C. and Burge, P. S. (1984) The sick building syndrome: prevalence studies. *Br. Med. J.* **289**, 1573–1575.

Chapter 17 / Physical Hazards

IONIZING RADIATIONS

Ionization is any process by which an atom or molecule loses or gains electrons, resulting in the production of electrically charged particles. Such particles are known as ions. Ionization is accompanied by a transfer of energy to the material in which the ions are formed. Certain radiations are capable of producing ionization. They are known as *ionizing radiations*.

Those for which standards of dosage are defined are alpha particles, beta particles, protons, neutrons, X-rays and gamma rays. The latter two are electromagnetic radiations similar to and propagated like light waves and radio waves, the remaining are material particles of atomic or subatomic size.

Occupational exposure results from work involving X-rays in industrial radiography or X-rays from radioactive isotopes in non-destructive testing, nuclear power electrical generation and many other industrial processes.

Occupations involving exposure are covered by Ionizing Radiations (Sealed Sources) Regulations 1969, Ionizing Radiations (Unsealed Radioactive Substances) Regulations 1968 and the Nuclear Licensing Act, 1965.

These require a pre-employment medical examination (carried out by an Employment Medical Adviser or Appointed Doctor), which includes a full haematological examination.

The exposure of workers is monitored by the wearing of a film badge, and subsequent medical examinations are not required unless exposure in the previous 12 months has exceeded three-tenths of the permitted dose (usually 15mSv).

When overdosage accidentally occurs, a special examination is required, in which lymphocyte culture is undertaken and chromosomal abnormalities looked for. The percentage of abnormalities gives an index of exposure.

Units. The International System (SI) units are a consistent set of units for use in all branches of science. These have been adopted on the recommendation of the International Commission on Radiation Units and Measurement (ICRU).

The SI *Unit of Radioactivity* is the becquerel (Bq) which is equal to one nuclear transformation per second. ($3 \cdot 7 \times 10^{10}$ Bq = 1 Curie (Ci).)

The SI *unit of absorbed dose* is the gray (Gy) equal to one joule/kilogram (J/kg) (1Gy = 100 rad).

The SI *unit of dose equivalent* is the joule/kilogram (J/kg). On the recommendation of *ICRU* this unit is called the sievert (Sv). (1Sv = 100 rem.)

Quality Factor (Q). For determining dose limits for radiological protection purposes a modifying factor termed the quality factor (Q) is used to take account of the kind of radiation and so obtain the *dose equivalent*.
Dose equivalent (Sv) = Absorbed dose (Gy) × Quality Factor (Q).

Q = 1 for X-ray, and gamma rays and beta particles;

Q = 3 for thermal neutrons;

Q = 20 for alpha particles.

Biological Effects of Exposure to Ionizing Radiation

Very high doses of radiation can kill a cell, but lower doses can prevent a cell from dividing or can damage the genetic material contained in the nucleus causing it to divide abnormally.

The biological effects of exposure to ionizing radiation fall into two categories:

1. Somatic — effects which are manifest in the exposed individual.

2. Genetic — effects which occur in the reproductive cell and are manifest in the exposed individual's descendants.

Somatic effects on the fetus are sometimes wrongly confused with genetic effects. As well as an increased chance of childhood cancer, fetal irradiation can result in impairment of growth, microcephaly, mental retardation and other congenital defects.

Acute severe exposure results in the acute radiation syndrome — nausea, headache, anorexia, followed by a period of apparent well-being prior to the onset of vomiting, diarrhoea, epilation and fulminating infection due to the total destruction of the marrow and immune system.

Late effects of ionizing radiation exposure either to an acute over-exposure or to repeated small exposures, include cataract formation (stochastic effect) or the induction of cancer or genetic effects (non-stochastic). The larger the dose of radiation the more likely it is that the initiating event resulting in abnormal cells will occur. Thus for non-stochastic effects it is not the severity of the effect which is a function of radiation dose but the probability of its occurrence.

Internal irradiation of small areas of tissue or organs may result from the absorption of radioactive isotopes and deposition and concentration in specific tissues, e.g. radioactive iodine in thyroid, plutonium, radium and phosphorus in bone. Intense irradiation of tissues may result from such events and, depending on dose, may cause total destruction of tissue or may give rise to carcinogenesis in those organs.

NOISE

'Unwanted sound'. Exposure to noise causes:

1. Temporary deafness (temporary threshold shift) — directly related to exposure.

2. Permanent hearing loss after a variable period, when TTS becomes irreversible. Begins and is maximal at 4000 Hz.

Audiogram tracing with dip at 4000 Hz is characteristic of noise-induced deafness.

Loudness is related to the intensity of sound energy, and the decibel (dB) is the unit of measurement.

The decibel is a logarithmic unit showing the ratio between two different intensities. It is determined by multiplying by 10 the logarithm to the base 10 of the ratio:

$$\text{n dB} = 10 \log_{10} \frac{I_1}{1_2}$$

Thus a twofold increase in intensity means a difference in decibels of:

$10 \times \log_{10} 2 = 10 \times 0{\cdot}3010 = 3{\cdot}01$ dB;

a tenfold increase $= 10 \times \log_{10} 10 = 10$ dB;

a hundredfold increase: $10 \times \log_{10} 100 = 10 \times 2 = 20$ dB and so on.

In audiometry, the threshold of normal hearing is defined as 0 dB, which is equivalent to a sound pressure of 20 micropascals (μPa).

A whisper at 1 metre has an intensity of 30 dB; normal speech of 60 dB, and a shout 90 dB.

Frequency determines the pitch of sound, and is measured in Hertz, which are the number of cycles or double vibrations per second of the sound source. Middle C has a frequency of 256 Hz; doubling the frequency produces a note one octave higher.

Measurement. Noise level meters contain three circuits, A, B and C. A and B reduce sensitivity to lower frequencies and A measurements simulate human ear best. These are expressed as dBA.

Levels about 80 dBA indicate need for hearing protection.

Personal Protection. For levels between 80 and 100 dBA — glass down or moulded ear plugs.

For levels over 100 dBA, earmuffs with fluid-filled seals.

Audiometry. There are differing views on the value of audiometry in hearing conservation. On the one hand, it has been said with truth that it has never prevented deafness; on the other hand, routine audiometry in noisy occupations gives some indication of the effectiveness of preventive measures, and a pre-employment audiogram gives a base-line against which subsequent hearing loss can be compared.

Audiometry records hearing thresholds for pure tone notes over a range of frequencies from ½ to 8 kHz. Testing should be carried out in a sound-proof booth, as extraneous noise is liable to affect the subject's response. It is recommended that ideally subjects should not have been exposed to loud noise for 48 hours before testing, to avoid the effects of temporary threshold shift; this may be a counsel of perfection, but at least there should have been no exposure on the day of testing.

The classic pattern of the audiogram in noise-induced deafness shows a dip or notch in the tracing at 4 kHz; but interpretation is not always easy, particularly when there is also conductive deafness, and in older subjects where the expected effects of presbycusis on the thresholds for higher frequencies have to be taken into account. If there is a hearing loss of more than 90 dB in the 4, 6 and 8 kHz bands, the dip or notch will of course not have been seen because there will be no tracing for these frequencies.

For standardized techniques of audiometry and classification of hearing loss in industry, *see* HSE Discussion Document *Audiometry in Industry* (1979).

Some countries require regular audiograms for workers exposed to defined noise levels at annual intervals, or even more often. In Britain, the Health and Safety Executive *recommends* it for workers exposed to 105 dB or over, but makes no mention of frequency. An EEC Committee is now (1984) proposing regular audiometry for all workers exposed to 85 dB and over.

Claims for Benefit. Occupational deafness is a Prescribed Industrial Disease (No. 48) in certain specified noisy occupations involving use of pneumatic percussive tools, and in drop forging.

Successful claimants must have worked for at least 10 years in one or more of the following occupations, and in the 5 years before the claim:

a. Work wholly or mainly in rooms or sheds where there are machines engaged in weaving man-made or natural (including mineral) fibres or on the bulking-up of fibres in textile manufacturing.

b. The use of chain-saws in forestry.

c. The use of, or work in the immediate vicinity of, pneumatic percussive tools used: (1) on metal; (ii) for drilling rock in quarries or underground; (iii) in mining coal; for at least an average of one hour per working day.

AND occupations involving the use of any of the following tools or machinery, or work wholly or mainly in the immediate vicinity of them:

d. Pneumatic percussive tools or high-speed grinding tools in the cleaning, dressing or finishing of cast metal or of ingots, billets or blooms.

e. Pneumatic percussive tools on metal in the shipbuilding or ship-repairing industries.

f. Drop-forging plant (including plant for drop-stamping or drop-hammering) or forging press plant engaged in the shaping of metal.

g. Certain machines engaged in wood-working.

h. Machines engaged in cutting, shaping or cleaning metal nails.

i. Plasma spray guns engaged in the deposition of metal.

To qualify for benefit, there must be an average hearing loss of 50 dB in both ears due to inner ear damage, which in at least one ear is deemed to be due to noise at work.

References

Beagley H. A. and Barnard S. (1982) *Manual of Audiometric Techniques*. Oxford Medical Publications. Oxford University Press.

Bryan and Tempest W. (1980) *Industrial Audiometry*. 2nd ed. Audiology Group, Electrical Engineering Department, University of Salford.

*VIBRATION**

The best recognized disorder associated with the use of vibrating tools is 'white finger' or 'dead hand' — the Raynaud phenomenon, which is intermittent pallor or cyanosis of the fingers without clinical evidence of blockage of the large vessels.

The vibration frequencies most likely to cause trouble lie within the range of 40–125 Hz.

Decalcification of the carpal bones, and osteoarthritis of arm joints, especially the elbows, are long-term effects.

Russian workers have reported similar phenomenon in the feet in workers standing for long periods where vibro thickeners are used in the mixing of ferroconcrete panels. They say that these vibrations also cause headaches, vertigo, nausea and vomiting by their action on the vestibular apparatus. Other workers report that whole body vibration can cause motion sickness, blurred vision, loss of efficiency and discomfort. The body may amplify vibrations of certain frequencies because of natural resonance.

Preventive measures include the wearing of suitable warm clothing, including gloves; frequent short breaks in the use of the tool, rather than less frequent longer ones; and proper maintenance of tools. With some tools it is possible to devise anti-vibration mountings; the application of engineering ingenuity will produce a number of ways of controlling exposure.

Reference

Gierke H. E. and Nixon C. W. (1976) Effects of intense infra-sound on man. In: Tempest W. (ed.) *Infra-sound and Low Frequency Vibration*. London, Academic Press, pp. 115–47.

* Taylor W., Pearson J., Kell R. L. and Keighley J. D. (1971) Vibration syndrome in forestry commission chain-saw operators. *Br. J. Ind. Med.* **28**, 83–89; Grebenjuk V. P. The Effect of Vibration on the Human Body. Royal Aircraft Establishment. Library Translation No. 1611.

HEAT AND COLD

Difficult to defined acceptable standards because of individual variations in tolerance and body's ability to acquire a degree of tolerance to temperatures outside normal range. Temperatures of 18·3–21·1 °C (65–70 °F) with good ventilation usually regarded as comfortable for sedentary or light work, 12·8–15·6 °C (55–60 °F) for heavy work — with humidity within range 30–60%.

Where working conditions are necessarily hot and artificial cooling impracticable, protective clothing (perhaps ventilated) is required. If the wearing of this is impracticable, duration of exposure must be limited. Similar considerations apply in reverse to work in extreme cold.

Heat Illness. For a description of body heat production and loss, and protection against excessive heat, *see* pp. 52–3.

1. Heat syncope. Giddiness, acute physical fatigue or collapse may occur due to exercise, without lack of water or salt.

2. Water depletion heat exhaustion. Thirst, fatigue, giddiness, fever and delirium may arise from inadequate replacement of water lost in sweating.

3. Salt depletion and heat cramps. Fatigue, giddiness, nausea, vomiting and painful muscle spasms (miner's cramp) occur in men doing heavy physical work in heat, when sweating excessively, drinking a lot of water but not replacing salt.

4. Prickly heat. Rash and prickling sensations in hot, humid weather when the skin is wet with sweat.

5. Heat stroke. If the body cannot prevent temperature rise, in exposure to intense heat or during exercise in less severe heat, a coma will occur. It will be fatal unless the victim is cooled rapidly.

Cold. When working outside in cold climates workers should be protected with suitable clothing. Protective clothing should also be worn by workers who have to enter deep freeze plants, for example for food storage. The rapid expansion of air from the exhaust of a pneumatic tool can cause freezing. It is unlikely that the worker would continue to hold this long enough for frostbite to occur, but the cooling can be sufficient to freeze the glove to the tool. This extreme chilling will enhance the effects of vibration white finger.

Immersion hypothermia. Accidental immersion in water can cause rapid chilling which can be fatal within a few minutes. Where accidental immersion can occur workers should be protected with suitable warm clothing and buoyancy aids.

Sea Surface	*Temperature*	*Maximum Time of Immersion for Survival*
0 °C	(32 °F)	¼ hour
2½ °C	(36½ °F)	½ hour
5 °C	(41 °F)	1 hour
10 °C	(50 °F)	3 hours
15 °C	(59 °F)	7 hours
20 °C	(68 °F)	16 hours
25 °C	(77 °F)	3 days or more

After rescue, rapid rewarming in hot water is the accepted practice for young healthy subjects. In babies and the elderly, who may suffer from chronic hypothermia, gradual rewarming is preferable.

NON-IONIZING RADIATIONS

Lasers. A laser is an electro-optical device for concentrating visible light (wave lengths 10^3–10^4 Ångstrom units) into a narrow beam of intensely high energy. These beams may be continuous or pulsed (intermittent).

They are used in micro-welding and precision measurement of machine tools, in range finding and night flying, and new applications are continually being found.

Hazards. The laser beam can cause heating and destruction of tissues. The eye is particularly vulnerable, and damage to the lens and retinal burns may occur. The degree of damage depends on the wave length of the light and its energy. Recommended maximum exposures for a pulse duration of 10^{-6}–10^{-2} seconds are 10^{-8} joule/cm^2 at the front of the eye, or 10^{-2} joule/cm^2 calculated at the retina.

Control
    Eye protection.
    Enclosure of working area and restriction of numbers allowed therein.

Reduction of reflective surfaces within working area.

Warning signal when beam switched on.

Full ophthalmic examination before beginning the work, repeated after any incident which could cause eye damage. (It is probably wise to exclude those with monocular or virtually monocular vision.)

A Code of Practice for the use of laser systems was produced by the Ministry of Technology (now Department of Trade and Industry) in 1969.

Ultraviolet Light. Radiations with wave length 10^2–10^4 Ångstrom units. Produced by carbon arc, tungsten and mercury vapour lamps, welding arcs and metals heated over 3000 °C.

Hazards. Arc eye, conjunctivitis and keratitis. Permanent damage unlikely. Treated by instillation of 1 in 1000 adrenaline.

Erythema and burning of skin.

Infrared Radiation. Radiation of wave length 10^4–10^7 Ångstrom units. Work with sources of intense heat may produce anterior cortical cataract.

MICROWAVES

Very high frequency radio waves with wavelengths of from 1 mm to 1 m. The energy causes vibration of molecules (heat) but is insufficient to cause ionization. The lens is particularly vulnerable (cataract) as it cannot dissipate heat through increasing blood supply. The suggested maximum permissible exposure is a field with a power density of 0·01 watt/cm^2 (Medical Research Council).

The power density of emission from microwave ovens should not exceed 5 milliwatts/cm^2 at any point 5 cm or more from the external surface of the appliance (British Standard 5175).

PRESSURE

Tunnelling under water and diving, or work in diving bells, entail exposure to hyperbaric pressures.

Compression may cause pain in ears and sinuses — possibly rupture of eardrums.

The Diving Operations Special Regulations (1960) require a six-monthly medical examination by EMAS or Appointed Doctor. The Submarine Pipelines (Diving Operations) Regulations (1976), Off-Shore Installations (Diving Operations) Regulations (1974) and Merchant Shipping (Diving Operations) Regulations (1975) require a more stringent annual examination by a specially authorized doctor.

Decompression Sickness. Too rapid decompression leads to formation of bubbles of nitrogen from bloodstream which has dissolved at higher pressures. Symptoms ('bends') depend on site of bubbles.

Acute. Limb pains and itching. Vomiting and dizziness. Tingling or paralysis of limbs. Dyspnoea. Headache and bizarre visual symptoms. Angina, collapse, coma and death.

Chronic. Paralysis. Aseptic bone necrosis.

Rate of decompression specified by Regulations. Pre-employment examinations and monthly re-examinations statutory, together with examination on return from illness or injury.

Similar symptoms may occur in flying at very high altitudes. Prevented by breathing pure oxygen at ground level before ascent.

The taking of accurate measurements of the working environment is part of the specialist field of the occupational hygienist. New methods and refinements are being developed rapidly, and details of sampling equipment would not be appropriate in a book of this kind.

However, some mention of devices available for preliminary field work must be made. The most generally useful are detection tubes, which are available for a wide range of chemicals. These consist of a silica gel coated with the appropriate reagent, which produces a colour change. The length of tube for which this change extends gives a rough indication of the concentration of the contaminant, after the drawing of a measured volume of air into the tube by a hand pump. (The 'breathalyser' used as a screening test for car drivers who have taken alcohol is an example.) The best known are those made by Drager, but other companies also manufacture them.

Smoke tubes provide an indication of the efficacy of exhaust ventilation, and the Tyndall effect (rendering visible otherwise invisible dust particles by means of scattered light projected from a suitable source) can reveal the presence of dust which would not otherwise be apparent in a working environment.

More accurate quantitative measurements of atmospheric contaminants will not normally be carried out by the industrial physician. Many direct reading instruments are available which depend on some physical property of the contaminant. Personal samplers which can be worn by selected workers collect material over a measured period for subsequent analysis, and gravimetric samplers can be installed at fixed points for the same purpose.

Dust samplers are now available which carry devices for selecting ranges of particle size at their inlets. These contain membrane filters and are fitted with battery-driven pumps. Another instrument is the thermal precipitator, which draws dust-laden air down a vertical passage and along a horizontal channel containing a glass slide, on to which particles are precipitated partly by gravity and partly thermally by a heated wire. The konimeter, an instrument in which a small volume of air impinged on a jelly-coated glass slide, has proved inaccurate, and is now rarely used.

The thermal environment and humidity are measured by wet and dry bulb thermometers. Humidity is calculated by reference to charts. The Kata thermometer, available in three temperature ranges, takes account of air velocity.

Noise meters measure the sound pressure level and the frequency distribution. The 'A' weighting element, which is that normally used in environmental surveys is designed for the frequencies perceptible to the human ear.

References

Methods for the Detection of Toxic Substances in Air. Some 325 booklets produced by the Health and Safety Executive, available from Government Bookshops (*see* pp. 133–4).

Occupational Hygiene. An Introductory Guide. Jones, Hutcheson and Dymott (1981). London, Croom Helm.

Schilling R. S. F. (ed.) (1973) *Occupational Health Practice.* London, Butterworth, Ch. 13, 14, 15.

Index